Finding Joy in Sorrow

Finding Joy in Sorrow

JUDY VOSS

Finding Joy In Sorrow
©2022, 2017, 2014 by Judy Voss

Cover photo by ©Benoit Daoust/123Rf.com
Printed in the United States of America

Library of Congress Cataloging-in-Publication Data:
Finding Joy In Sorrow/Judy Voss
ISBN – 13:978-1500246815; ISBN-10:1500246816
1. End of life 2. Death and dying 3. Hospice care 4. Angels

The true stories contained in FINDING JOY IN SORROW
may seem familiar to the reader as these events do occur
frequently in living and dying. Some of the stories have had
names or details changed to protect the privacy and
confidentiality of those involved.
This book is not intended to be a substitute for medical or legal
advice and encourages readers to seek professional counsel.

Scripture quotations are taken from the *New Living
Translation* Holy Bible, Copyright © 1996, 2004.
Used by permission of Tyndale House Publishers, Inc.,
Wheaton, Illinois 601689. All right reserved.

Dedication

This book is dedicated to my dad, Carlton Fairchild, who stepped into heaven on May 10, 2022. The countless patients I have cared for throughout my nursing career taught me far more than what I learned from textbooks and teachers, and they are who enabled me to care for Dad despite my sorrow.

Dad's death and dying story is woven throughout this book because he is ultimately my reason for writing it.

Joy: *an especially ecstatic or exultant happiness for someone or something greatly valued or appreciated*

Sorrow: *a feeling of sadness or grief caused especially by the loss of someone or something*

Author's Note

Joy... such a tiny word that can brighten any moment of any day and is capable of holding our most treasured memories.

Yet joy seems so remote when sorrow consumes us, whether due to a loved one's death, a horrific tragedy, or a severe loss such as a divorce, a job, or our home. Sorrow comes in all sizes and disguises, creeping up on you slowly or with an unsuspecting wallop that will knock you to your knees, wrench you of your sleep, steal your peace of mind, and fracture your heart. It may leave you exposed and vulnerable to anything and everything.

But hopefully joy will return. Whether it taps you intermittently on your shoulder or drops plainly in your lap, joy can wiggle its way back into your life, your memories, and your heart.

My prayer is that these true stories of death, dying, and living through grief will bring you a peace that passes all understanding when sorrow steps across your threshold... and you can find joy in the midst of your sorrow.

Judy Voss

Finding Joy In Sorrow

Contents

Dedication
Author's Note

1 Language of Death

Because death and dying have long been a taboo subject, it has been laden with its own language of avoidance through the use of euphemisms or slang words. We use gentler words because they are less threatening and provide some distancing of death before the full impact can be grasped or comprehended. Especially with children, words should be chosen carefully so as not to convey one who has died as being *asleep* or *lost* which would add more confusion and distress for the child.

Whatever the age of the one approaching death, each conveys very similar desires:

> **1.** *To maintain relationships with those who are special in their lives and perhaps with those who have become estranged.*
> **2.** *To know who will care for them in their last months, days, or hours.*
> **3.** *To listen carefully to their requests and maintain their dignity at all times.*
> **4.** *To be honest and open with them.*
> **5.** *To be touched.*
> **6.** *To be allowed closure and time to say goodbye*

We Gotta' Talk

Why are we hesitant to talk about what is probably going to be a natural, peaceful, and anticipated death? Why can't we honestly and openly discuss, until absolutely necessary, the deathbed scene that is generally tucked behind closed doors?

Perhaps we are afraid. Perhaps our denial has overtaken the obvious. Of course, we don't want our loved one to die as even the thought of being without them consumes us. But we still need to talk to them about death, even if we don't want to, for their sake and our own.

We must unlock those heavy doors of silence at the deathbed so we feel comfortable enough to crawl over side rails and around medical equipment (with approval, if needed) to hold and cuddle our loved ones. If that isn't possible, then simply sit at their bedside and hold their hand even though they may not have the strength to hold yours.

Then you must listen carefully. Did your loved one whisper something to you that you may not have heard from a distance? Did they tell you what they want sung at their funeral or where those important papers are? Did they tell you that they only have a few hours or few days before their death? Did they convey to you what their greatest needs and concerns are? You mustn't wait too long to listen as they may never repeat what you may have missed.

You may think the dying don't realize what is happening, but they most likely do. They are just afraid to broach such a tender topic for you and them... so help them. Now is the time to talk, and listen, because you may never have another opportunity.

Wiggle your Toes!

My hospice co-worker and Vietnam veteran Vickie could not communicate anything as she lay in her hospital bed connected to a ventilator that made rhythmic whooshing sounds that provided her a means of breathing. Her eyes were closed and her body still, except for the steady rising and falling of her chest due to her ventilator.

I patiently sat vigil at Vickie's bedside holding her hand, wishing she would return the gentle squeeze I occasionally gave hers. Staring closely at her face, I watched for a raise of her eyebrow or a twitch of her lips. Even a grimace would be welcome, anything to signal she was aware of her surroundings. No response came.

After a bit, I needed to stretch my legs so I slowly rose from my chair and walked softly alongside her hospital bed. As I inched closer to the foot of her bed, I slid my hand along the side rail.

When I approached the end of Vickie's bed, I very gently swept my fingertips over the sheet that lay atop her toes. To my great surprise, the sheet gently moved below my fingertips!

Startled, I quickly lifted my hand from atop the sheet, stopped in my tracks, and looked in awe to Vickie who still lay motionless with her eyes closed and face and body relaxed, still breathing with the assistance of her ventilator. I thought I must have been imagining things so I tenderly laid my hands on the sheet that covered her feet and asked her to wiggle her toes… and she did! I cannot explain, ever, how shocked I was but so amazed and grateful to know she absolutely could hear me and had the ability to communicate by wiggling her toes!

Within minutes, her family and pastor arrived and I shared my discovery, then Vickie acknowledged their presence by "answering" through her toes. What an amazing gift that Vickie was able to give even though it lasted for a very brief time!

So sadly, this valiant woman in the prime of her life, this American hero who died from exposure to Agent Orange while battling for freedom for those in an unknown land, died within hours of blessing us with her awareness. But we were so thankful that Vickie heard all the loving words, the prayers, and scripture read to her in her final time on earth.

Vickie taught me a very, very powerful lesson in listening well, without my ears, and I will forever be grateful to her.

Adjusting our Attitude

The avoidance of discussing death and dying may be related to our fears of the unknown. The uncertainties can be many such as the anticipation of suffering or pain, concerns over one's dignity being maintained, wondering if death will come suddenly or as a result of a tragedy, during sleep or in wakefulness, will death occur at home, will death come when we are alone, will we be in a comatose or vegetative state, and/or will concerns of life after death or any unfinished business impede the hope of having a peaceful death.

Perhaps we hold onto the thought that we may be the first immortal one and so death is not of any concern, which is certainly classified as *death denying*. If we don't talk about it then it won't happen, right? Wrong.

Dixie and Ray

After ringing the doorbell, a shaky voice from deep inside the home yelled, "Come in!"

After pushing the door open, I spoke out, "It's Judy from hospice." I could hear the familiar rumble of an oxygen machine and my eyes automatically looked at the floor where the oxygen tubing was easy to spot against an old green, shag carpet.

As I followed the snake-like pathway, my steps led me to a bedroom in the west side of the home. The setting sun filled the room, spilling onto my patient lying in the hospital bed.

"I'm so glad you came," the weak voice of my dying patient said. Behind the whisper lay a frail lady named Dixie who had fought long and hard against lung cancer. Her disease had weakened her body but not her wonderful spirit for living.

"Hi, Dixie. What a gorgeous, sunny day," I said.

"Yes, it was until I fell," she whispered.

Just then Ray, Dixie's husband, entered our little world of sunshine. "She sure took a tumble!" Ray exclaimed. "I found her on the kitchen floor. She's never fallen like that before."

My heart started to squeeze as I was aware that certain facts would need to be discussed before I left Dixie and Ray. They both said nearly in unison, "Please tell us both what to expect. We've always been up front and honest with each other."

After a tearful discussion about the expectations of Dixie's decline, as she grew closer to death, Ray accompanied me to the front door I had entered an hour earlier. As we walked along the snake-like path, Ray told me how much in love he and Dixie were, "Even after all these years we make every moment as happy as we can. We love to laugh even when times are tough."

My patient and her loved one encouraged me, reminding me that there are lots of good times despite the bad, there's joy to be found in sorrow. Every moment of every day is to be savored and shared, they reminded me.

Can you hold me?

During one of my hospice visits, I discovered that what we think is the obvious problem…isn't. That's what Lucy taught me.

"Can you hold me?" The words were barely audible. I had never been asked that by a stranger or patient before, so I asked Lucy to please repeat what she said just in case I misunderstood her. The words again were just barely audible, "Can you hold me?" Then Lucy tried to lean forward in her bed for me to gently reach around her frail body, a body that would soon be held by one much greater than I.

I wrapped my arms around Lucy's shoulders very gently, so I would not hurt her or hinder her already labored breathing. Her body felt like a wounded little bird whose love for flying had vanished. What I desired to do was to pick Lucy up and place her in the arms of the One waiting for her, but sometimes He asks for a little more patience from us. As I held Lucy, I silently prayed for her to sleep in peace and to be free from the pain that had so fiercely dwelt inside her for so long.

Then my thoughts turned to Lucy's family and the hundreds of others who attend to their dying loved ones hour after hour, day after day, and month after month, despite the sadness that engulfs them. Their strength amazes me and when they say to me, "I don't know how you can do your job!" I explain to them that what they are doing is a much greater sacrifice and done with a love stronger than any other. They are the ones who deserve the praise, as there is no greater marathon in life than attending to a dying loved one. Please try to be there.

Listen up!

Our ears provide us a very powerful tool. By listening well we can learn volumes that may be vital in meeting the needs of the dying and recognizing their moment of passing. One of my very intuitive gentlemen wanted to remind his family how certain he was that he would not see another tomorrow. Just before he took his last breath he said, "It is time to separate now," and he did.

In Pope John Paul II's book *Be Not Afraid!* he said he was intimidated by human suffering and was at one time afraid to approach the dying.

Just like Pope John Paul II, I have also been afraid to approach the dying at many times in my life, especially as a young nurse. It was obvious in the hospital where the dying lay because their door was usually closed far enough so no one could peek in and see what approaching death looks like. If the door wasn't ajar, often the curtain was pulled so the patient lay in total isolation, out of view of any passerby.

We must recognize that the dying certainly have special needs and we must do all we can to fulfill them, which includes touching them without wavering.

One of the most humbling moments of touch for me is when I take hold of my patient's hand and the only way they can communicate with me is through a return squeeze. I can discover a lot from that first squeeze, as I did one day when I stepped into Joe's hospital room. He didn't turn his head to look at me as I sat at his bedside, looking intently at him. The white linens remained unwrinkled about his body as he lay perfectly still in his hospital bed. The sterile air was silent except for the TV monitor, which was shouting cartoon gibberish into his left ear. I quickly reached for the monitor, lowered the volume, and changed the channel to quiet and calming music.

Upon taking Joe's right hand in mine and quietly speaking his name, I expected him to open his eyes and greet me as many of my patients do. However, that wasn't to be. But I was pleasantly and thankfully surprised to see a pair of gray, bushy eyebrows rise up slightly in awareness and acknowledgement of my greeting and touch. Instead of speaking, Joe clenched my hand in his with all the strength a hefty-looking man like him could clench.

With more enthusiasm, I said again, "Hi, Joe!"

Then Joe raised our joined hands slightly off his bed. What a strong healthy grip he had, at least in this hand, while his left hand lay paralyzed at his side. It was as if I could feel the fear Joe felt inside, which he silently expressed as his fingers tightly encircled mine.

Because I feel it is so important to be open and honest with my patients, I asked Joe if he knew he had had a stroke, and with that he released and then squeezed my hand again, with greater strength than before. I slowly and calmly shared with Joe what I knew he could expect regarding his care in the near future. Joe tightened his grip and then would slightly relax it, acknowledging awareness. Thankfully, his face showed no fear or pain.

With eyes now slightly open and peeking at me, I continued to share with Joe what I knew would bring him comfort and ease his fear and anxiety of the unknown.

Through my misty eyes, I also shared what I experienced with others regarding the presence of angels and told him that when he is afraid they can comfort him. As my words rolled off my tongue, Joe's grip on my hand eased entirely for the first time during our visit.

Upon ending our time together and saying my good-byes, which included a kiss on Joe's forehead, I promised him I would call his sister who lived an hour away and let her know how he was doing, as she also was in her eighties and very concerned about her little brother.

Joe's sister was so disappointed she was unable to get a ride to see him that day or the next, but she was so very glad and relieved to hear about my response from Joe. The report that was conveyed to her regarding his condition was that he was totally unresponsive and would probably not realize her presence if she were with him. Oh, my, I clarified that was not true at all!

My very first stroke patient, who was just like Joe, was my Grandpa Vincent. He had a severe stroke the morning I left for my first day of college in 1971. Grandpa's only source of transport for thirteen years was by wheelchair. The only thing Grandpa could say after his stroke was, "Good for a Republican!" (Amen to that, Grandpa!) He was able to communicate many memorable things through his body language, especially through the squeeze of his hand. I will tell of his miracle later.

Lock it Up

Sometimes just being present and sharing special moments in silence is enough. Kathy Sullivan explains it best:

What a guy! I met Stephen while working the evening shift as an Administrative Secretary in the Hospice Care Center. Stephen was a resident of Washington D.C. but, because of his terminal condition, he moved closer to his family in Florida and eventually spent his last days at the Care Center. Stephen was a kind, soft-spoken, intelligent young man who studied and taught Shakespeare in Washington before he became ill.

Every evening, at about the same time, Stephen would slowly walk to the nurses' station with his cane in hand, stand in the doorway and ask me, "Is it time to lock the front door yet?" I was the person that locked the door every evening to ensure the Care Center staff knew what visitors desired entry after hours. This ritual continued every night until the time came that Stephen was too weak to take our memorable nightly walk.

I learned an unforgettable lesson during Stephen's stay at the Care Center that taking those leisurely walks to lock the front door each night was not about locking the front door at all.

When Children Talk, You Better Listen

Our children can teach us immeasurable things if we heed their words. There are books full of stories told by children who have envisioned and predicted their death with pure certainty and a calm acceptance. One such book is *A Window To Heaven* by Diane M. Komp, M.D., who is a pediatric oncologist. Her little patients, who were faced with dying, expressed to her a great comfort in an understanding of better life hereafter, a life they anticipated spending with Jesus. Dr. Komp heeded the words her children shared with her when they voiced the timeliness of their death, which helped her reclaim her own faith, and became a better listener and believer of little ones.

Truth Telling or Not

Whether we realize it or not, there are certain ways we tend to communicate, or not communicate, sad or happy news to others. Perhaps for a period of time we choose to keep secret an anticipated divorce, a probable job change, a move away from our parents, or a loss of income. We may prolong keeping these secrets for various reasons but generally it is to protect others from premature or potential sadness or grief.

There is much we can learn from those who are dying by the way they communicate to us. If we pay close attention to what they say, hear, or see we may discover they have a clear understanding of their approaching death. Some have predicted the hour and day they will die with amazing accuracy.

Many who are approaching death have an awareness of their final days and hours and may even sense or envision the presence of their deceased loved ones, angels, or other celestial presence. This understanding is known as *Near Death Awareness*.

Not everyone believes that death should be openly discussed as Sociologists Barney Glaser and Anselm Strauss have discovered. They address four styles of communication that are specific to death and dying, which they discuss in their book *Awareness of Dying*.

The first communication style is called *closed awareness* where others may know about one's approaching death but the one dying is purposely not informed. Some feel that decisions regarding medical care should be decided on by the family so patient involvement and their awareness of their own death is not believed essential. Others may feel it is the will of God to let an illness progress so the information is not shared with the afflicted.

The second style of communication is known as *suspected awareness* where the ill person may sense their death approaching but it is still not openly discussed or verified by others. Perhaps loved ones of the dying feel it is best that the very ill not be burdened with sad news prematurely.

Next is *mutual pretense* where everyone, including the dying, is aware of one's approaching death but the subject is still avoided. Some feel that talking about death or beginning hospice care may cause death to transpire earlier or diminish any hope of remission. This style is similar to the adage of having an elephant in your living room yet everyone avoids talking about something so obvious. Dying is generally not a secret to the dying, even if others think it is. Just ask them and they will tell you so.

Finally, with *open awareness* an honest discussion of an approaching death between the dying, their loved ones, their caregivers and any others involved in end of life decisions is permissible and encouraged. This style allows the sharing of needs and concerns of the dying and of those who provide care, plus it provides time for closure and completion of life's details that may not have been addressed. In families with estranged loved ones, this extra time allows an opportunity to reunite and make amends. Another advantage of *open awareness* is the opportunity to complete Advance Directives, which are discussed later in this book.

As a caregiver, it is imperative that one recognizes that certain cultures may have their own style of communication that may not allow open discussion of death and dying. It is with respect that caregivers must honor these requests of silence and deliver compassionate and nonjudgmental care to all. Jake and Elisabeth, a couple I refer to later, used *open awareness* throughout his illness, as that is what they practiced throughout their marriage. Jake received hospice care for four months so many of his and his families' anxieties were addressed early on. Their open communication allowed their adult children time for visits and to assist in his care giving, plus it provided Jake a peace of mind in knowing that his wife would be well cared for after his death.

Life Review

A very important part of bringing closure to one's purpose in living is through telling stories from the past, even going back to their earliest memories, reviewing all of their life. I never imagined that I would be honored to attend to true war heroes, volunteers from numerous organizations, those who have given so generously to the needy, as well those who were far less privileged. No matter who we are or what we have been, each of us has certain needs when death approaches…one of great importance is to find a purpose in living.

Our Life's Book

Our life is like a book. Some of us have a chapter or two we would like to erase or do-over but that's life. We are only human. Our autobiography is unique to ourselves, some with much greater length than others and some are sadly way too short.

We cannot deceive our body into thinking we can live years longer by looking younger than our numbered years, no matter how much plastic surgery we have (and I could use some), how many vitamins we take, or how many miles we walk, run, or bike. We must all one day look death squarely in the face and say, "OK, I am now ready for you. I know what to expect, and I will not be afraid."

It is now time to take the next brave step into discovering what dying was like for those I have cared for. My prayer is you will gain a greater appreciation for living by sharing in the lives of the dying and those who compassionately and joyously cared for them.

Please remember that each story you read and each sign or symptom that has occurred is unique to each individual. Some concerns or needs may not transpire at all. Always remember your doctor and/or hospice team are great resources for you. You will soon learn much more about hospice.

2 Angels and Other Things

Angel feathers, sensing or seeing angels, visions of heaven and those who have passed, a miracle healing, a light surrounding an accident survivor, and an encounter with Jesus are all bits of stories told by people I know or met during my forty years of nursing. While we may not be able to scientifically explain or prove these events, they did happen and has assured me there is life after our earthly death, commonly referred to as *afterlife.*

Throughout my nursing career, patients and their loved ones often asked if I believe in heaven and in angels. Yes, I do, and I have my own angel feather and stories to prove it! In the thousands of hospice patients' homes I entered, many displayed pictures or figurines of Jesus, of angels, and the holy family and found comfort in sharing their beliefs and their stories, also.

Hospital Angels

Hospitals seem to have lots of great stories within their walls that attest to angels' existence. This story, told by a hospice co-worker and dear friend Cheryl Maxwell, strengthens that belief:

While working at the local hospital on the 3-11 shift, I had the pleasure to take care of an elderly gentleman in his nineties. Mr. Brown was deeply religious and read his Bible frequently. I had been his nurse for several days but on this particular day he had received the results of all the cardiac tests he had undergone.

He stated, "Well, did you hear the news? They say my heart is shot and there's nothing more they can do for me." He then stated, "…but that's ok. I've lived a good, long life and I'm getting tired."

I tried to give him as much encouragement and support as I could.

At 10:00pm I was standing at my medication cart outside his room when out of the corner of my eye I saw two extremely tall, handsome men dressed in suits walk up to me. I was startled to see them because visiting hours were over at 8:00pm and all the doors except the Emergency Room door (where Security Guards sit) are locked. The two asked very politely if Mr. Brown was in room 521.

I told them yes, he was, and asked how they got upstairs without a security escort at this time of night.

One of the men just smiled and said, "We just walked right in; no one tried to stop us." They said they were from a local church and had heard Mr. Brown was here and wanted to visit him.

I asked Mr. Brown if he would accept visitors, and he said he would.

They walked to his bedside while I returned to my medicine cart outside his door. I heard them read scripture and pray with Mr. Brown.

Approximately ten minutes later, they walked out of the room, said "Thank you," and started walking back down the long hallway from which they came. I turned my head for a second to sign off a medication and when I looked up they were gone. I thought to myself that they might have gone into another patient's room so I hurried down the hall checking the rooms. I went straight to the desk that sits directly in front of the elevator and stairs. The

Charge Nurse and the secretary both reported seeing no visitors. Security was called and he also reported seeing no men of that description enter or leave the hospital that night.

I hurried down to Mr. Brown's room. He was still awake reading his Bible. I asked him if he had known the two men who had visited him.

He said, "No, but I greatly appreciated their visit because they had given me such peace."

I told him about the men literally vanishing and no one else in the hospital had seen them but him and me. I told Mr. Brown, "I think we just saw two angels." Mr. Brown only smiled and said nothing.

Mr. Brown was discharged before I arrived the next day. I heard he passed away two weeks later at home.

A Sleepy Caregiver

After hospice nurse Linda Neider arrived at her patient's home, she overheard the patient's niece apologizing to her aunt for falling asleep in the night and leaving her alone.

The aunt replied as she pointed to an empty chair in the corner, "I was not alone. That nice lady with the silver hair was here all night!"

As you guessed, the chair was empty when Linda and the patient's niece glanced over to it.

A Boy and his Angel

In early January of 2014, I picked up my grandchildren from school, Jillian, age 10, and my grandson Liam, just shy of age 8. Liam couldn't get the

Finding Joy In Sorrow

words out fast enough to tell me about an angel he saw in his home the evening before.

"Gramma, I went into the kitchen last night to get a drink of water and outside the patio door was an angel! He had blue eyes like mine!"

I asked him what he was wearing and Liam said he was dressed in white and had a circle of light around his head.

"Then he just disappeared!" Liam said.

Liam can tell some tales but this was definitely not one. He was adamant at what he had seen and conveyed the exact circumstances to his dad and his grampa later that day.

Five months later, I tested Liam's memory about his angel visit and he relayed the exact same story. It is often told that children can see things with their young eyes, like angels, that adults can't.

I'm Not Crazy!

While sitting on his sun porch, my patient, John, and I were discussing his approaching death. He had a very stern and worried look on his face while addressing his immediate physical concerns.

While John's wife sat patiently to his left, I asked him if there was something else I could do for him. I listened and watched him very closely, sensing something must have been bothering him terribly because he became far more anxious and restless.

"Take me to the vet," John said.

"Take you where?" I asked.

"To the vet!" John shot back.

"Do you mean the veterans' hospital?" I asked.

His wife spoke up, "He means to the veterinarian."

"That's the only thing I need," John asserted. "To be put to sleep!"

I asked John if he was afraid of suffering and afraid of dying. His eyes filled with tears and he nodded *yes* as he tried to contain his sobs.

Together we talked about dying. Then I asked John if he had seen angels or his deceased parents or other loved ones who had died.

He hesitantly nodded *yes* again.

As I looked to John's left, his wife had a questioning look on her face. Then she asked John, "Why didn't you tell me that?"

"Because you would have thought I was crazy!" John quickly responded. So again, the door of honesty about death had been opened wide, and we shared stories of heaven and angels…and dying.

In the Way of Angels

Wally, age 78, lay in a light coma but he was still able to respond through the squeeze of his hand and with a sweet grin on his lips. No words ever left his lips in the eight hours I sat at his bedside during his last day of life.

As Wally's three adult children circulated through his bedroom, I learned many wonderful things about Wally. He was a widower and sorely missed his loving spouse, even after a dozen years without her. His family shared his tragedy of the death of his and his wife's infant daughter many years prior.

Wally's eldest son told of an experience that occurred the day prior to my arrival. He had just stepped into his father's bedroom and as he stood in the doorway his father said, "Son, you need to move. You're standing in her way!"

He asked his father, "Whose way am I standing in?"

Wally answered, "Your mother's, of course!"

Later in the same day, Wally's son had sat next to his father's bed in front of the closet door. Wally said, "Son you need to move. You are blocking your mother and sister!"

The only sister that could have possibly been spoken of was the infant who died many years prior.

Angels in the Corner

My little gray-haired lady was very close to dying and no longer able to speak. After assessing her then comforting her daughter about her mother's approaching death, I asked if her mom had visions of angels and she said, "Yes!"

She conveyed to me that one week prior her mother kept staring at the corner in her bedroom. I asked her what she was seeing. She said, "Angels!" So I asked her if they really wear white robes and she adamantly responded, "Of course, they do!"

Another patient and his wife had many gorgeous angel figurines in their home so I knew they believed in angels. The elderly gentleman I was caring for was unable to speak so his wife conveyed that he had seen twin angels standing in the corner of his bedroom just a few days before my visit.

He died very peacefully less than a week later.

Go Away!

A very loving wife relayed this story to me about her husband who was approaching death.

"When I woke in the morning there were two angels in white standing at the foot of my husband's and my bed. I couldn't see their faces clearly, nor did I see wings, yet I knew they were angels who had come to take my husband to heaven. I told them, 'No. Go away! I am not ready for you to take him.' Then they disappeared.

"Again, that afternoon, I saw them standing at the foot of the bed, and I repeated my same request. They thankfully disappeared again."

Three days later when the angels came again, they left with her husband who accompanied them to heaven.

Angels in the Night

An angel story I remember vividly from my own childhood occurred in the middle of the night while sleeping on the couch downstairs in our two-story farmhouse. There were only two reasons why I would have been downstairs. The first would have been because I wasn't feeling well and, secondly, there was a thunderstorm roaring through the northern Adirondack skies, during which Mom insisted all six of us children bunker down in the living room because *we* were scared. I was the only one in the living room at the time so I must have been sickly, not scared. Neither Mom nor Dad ever recalls me being very sick.

From outside, I heard hundreds of female voices singing, but without words. The voices were high pitched and very much in harmony with one another. There were no instruments only voices singing, "Ahhhhh…" which lasted ten to fifteen minutes in my child's memory.

I recall sticking my fingers in my ears to see if that made a difference in my sense of hearing. It did not. The only thing that I have heard since that sounded similar to my angels was a piece written by Antonio Vivaldi.

I still wonder nearly fifty years later why the angels were singing to me. Was I near dying? I certainly don't recall feeling that way. The angels' voices gave me an unbelievable comfort in hearing them, and I had no doubt they were singing to me, not to the rest of my family of eight, and probably not to the cows in the pasture. I still do not know why then and why me.

Please, God! Don't take her!

One of my greatest reminders of the presence of God in my life is marked in a little square on my yearly calendar where the words *Jillian '04* is written, the day a miracle happened in my home.

I always looked forward to Fridays because I got to entertain my grandchild, Jillian, who is now nineteen years old. Jilly is God's precious gift to my oldest son Jimmy. She loves life and fills every waking moment with lots of action, animation, and is a terrific dancer.

Jillian learned to walk at nine months of age and so had progressed into running most places a year later on December 4, 2004. She and I would often sit outside my front door on our bench, and she would intermittently play on the grass nearby or walk among the plants between our house and sidewalk. This day was no exception.

After resting very briefly on the bench next to me, Jilly scooted her little bottom off the seat and started walking down the cement sidewalk, then she suddenly took off on a run. When I cautioned her to walk instead, Jilly fell head-first onto the cement, striking the middle of her forehead. I immediately raced to her and scooped my little granddaughter of twenty-one-months into my arms and raced her to the kitchen to get ice.

While she was loudly crying with tears rolling down her cheeks, I applied ice to her forehead and spoke softly to her, and over several minutes she gradually calmed. I knew the importance of keeping her awake in case she had a concussion, so I took her into the bedroom where she often played. Within just a few minutes, her head collapsed onto my shoulder, and she was silent.

As I looked at Jilly, I saw that she was extremely pale, and her breathing was very shallow and slow. I could not stir her no matter what I did. She was truly a little limp doll. I knew that if Jilly declined any further I would need to call for emergency assistance.

I laid her on the bed so I could assess her more thoroughly, yet quickly, and noticed she was not breathing. I knew within minutes her heart would stop.

Just before I decided I would have to call 911 and begin rescue breathing on Jilly, I prayed fervently and passionately, "Dear God, please don't take Jilly! How will I ever tell Jimmy?"

Then, in a flash, a starburst of light came off of Jilly's chest and shot through the glass out the bedroom window! Jilly then opened her eyes and said, "Gam."

I said, "Hi, Jill." I was so choked up with gratitude to God as I picked my little miracle up and carried her to the rocking chair in our living room. Together we rocked and watched *Dora the Explorer*, as Jilly sang along with her favorite character. The huge boo-boo was still very prevalent on her forehead but, most importantly, the damage inside Jilly's head had been healed.

I was so flooded with emotion that I cried and cried and cried tears of joy and relief. When Jimmy came to pick up Jill I cried even more telling him what happened. I simply could not stop crying! Jimmy kept saying, "Mom, she's ok! You don't need to cry anymore!"

But I still did, and I still get choked up when I recall what God did. I am so grateful for His miracle of Jillian's healing. Miracles happen every day, even for a sinner such as me, so never doubt it can happen to you.

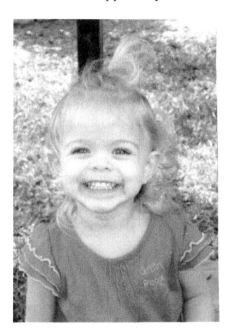

Jillian

Angels and Sunsets

Hospice volunteer Julie Eberhart Painter shares this awesome story of twin angels.

"Not all miracles are about winning the lottery or finding a cure for a terminal disease. Sometimes the miracle is gaining strength and dignity in the face of disaster, making a goal, or leaving a loving legacy.

"Our desire for miracles can get in the way of recognizing that God's way may be our best miracle. But now and then we get a really dramatic episode.

"One morning, I arrived at my volunteer coordinator's office, out of breath from a dash through the hot parking lot. She called, 'Come here a moment, Julie, I have a story to tell you.'

" 'That would be a switch,' I said. "I've shared enough stories with you.'

"Tears glittered in the corners of her eyes. 'We had a miracle here,' she began.

"Taking a seat, I settled in for the story."

'A couple of weeks ago when Mrs. Jones was dying, her family, about ten of them, gathered around her bed to say goodbye. Her son was having a hard time with his mother's impending death and needed to step outside onto the patio so she wouldn't see how upset he was. It was about eight o'clock, and the sun was beginning to set. Refreshed by the beauty of the sunset, he went to his car to get his camera and take a picture of the colorful display. When he returned, his mother had passed. He felt awful. He'd let her down.

'We tried to console him, explaining that often a dying person doesn't want to leave in front of his or her loved ones. He was not comforted and blamed himself. We could only hope he was resolving his guilt and processing his loss. Sadly, when his social worker called on him, he was still in complicated grief. She thought it would be a while before he came to terms with the fact that he couldn't have helped it and that it might have been her wish that he was outside just at that moment.

"Yesterday he burst through the door waving a large manila envelope. He pulled out two pictures and told us, 'I took these the night Mom passed away. I wanted you to have copies.' He spread the sunset pictures on my desk. At first, I couldn't believe it, but here it is. He gave me copies. Have a look for yourself.'

"She turned them around for me to see. As I looked at the pictures, I suddenly felt the hairs on the back of my neck rise. Two angels were posed on top of the sun. 'He'll be all right now,' I said.

"We don't often experience dramatic angel sightings. But we saw it in living color!"

A Bedroom Light

It was a very black night outside when I arrived at the home of my hospice patient who had died an hour prior. The family members were gathered in the master bedroom, some standing nearby and others sitting on the edge of the bed where their loved one laid. Each was tearful but accepting of the death of the ninety-year-old woman who had blessed their family for so many years.

While waiting for the funeral home director to arrive, the family and I remained at the bedside with the bedroom illuminated by a soft light positioned on the bedside table. The family shared in the woman's life review, reminiscing over some of the greatest joys she had brought them.

Once the funeral director arrived, he reviewed the family's funeral desires then he asked them to wait in another room while he and I prepared their loved one then transferred her to the stretcher. The family willingly obliged.

While assisting the director in gently lifting the lady up off her bed, the light in the bedroom went out! The room was suddenly pitch black and neither one of us could see a thing so we gently laid her back down on her bed we were braced against.

Just as soon as we laid her down, the light came back on. With pure puzzlement on both our faces, we proceeded to lift her again and the light went out again. Back down we laid her then we both straightened up from our crouched position wondering what we should do.

We decided that this woman must have a great sense of humor and acknowledged the same to her spirit! So we proceeded again to lift her and placed her on the stretcher without incident... and with a full lit room.

I Saw Angels

Joseph's eyes were wide open as they slowly followed something moving around his bed from the left side to the right. He had no fear in his face and didn't respond when I asked him what he saw.

It didn't take long to figure out what it may have been that Joseph was seeing. His mother, Maggie, explained, "Judy, there were three angels all dressed in white. I didn't see any wings but I know there were angels around my son's bed. I was watching them from across the room. I couldn't see their faces as their backs were to me. There was such a beautiful glow around them! No one believes me, but I know I saw them and I've seen them before today."

Another of my patients told me that for several days he had sensed angels around him as he sat in his recliner. He said that they gently bumped up against him. One angel placed a hand on his shoulder and he felt an immense warmth flood his body. He assured me he was on no medications, which some caregivers may say would explain what he felt. Without any doubt, I believed him. He died several days after sharing his angel story.

Guardian Angels

Try to recall an event that you wondered if an angel had something to do with your safety, an out of the ordinary event, or a quick healing. Did you ever say to yourself I wonder how in the world that happened? Ah! You may have encountered an angel on earth without realizing it.

On a shrine in St. Augustine, Florida, these words convey this belief the best, "…we do not see them, but they see us."

Billy Graham wrote in his book, *Angels: God's Secret Agents,* that *angels are real and that one day our eyes will be unscaled to see them.*

A Peek into Heaven

One of my greatest blessings has been standing, kneeling, or sitting at the bedside of the dying and having an awareness of heaven being very, very close to whomever I am caring for. I feel like I am on the edge of heaven, almost to the point of being able to glance in, my tippy toes on the verge of stepping over with them into afterlife. When I am at the bedside of the dying, I consider myself on sacred ground. I enter their home and their lives with reverence. To my patients and their loved ones, please know that it was an honor to be present for I was a stranger and you invited me into your lives.

The closest you will ever get to sensing heaven is by being present during those last hours and minutes before your loved one's death... so try to be there. You may also feel close enough to dip into that heavenly sea or perhaps skip along its shore, yet it is not your turn to play there just yet. But you can still share in your loved one's experience by talking about it and listening carefully to what they say. Then try imagining it as they describe it to you. What an opportunity you have!

Preparing for Heaven

As adults we know how we have lived our lives, what we have done and not done, what we have said and not said, so we should have a good sense of how God will judge us with regard to entering heaven. Even though we may have different styles of worship and wear different attire (or none at all), and the décor of our church might be different, all are the same if God is the center and we strive to be like Him.

If you have not read the book *Heaven is for Real* or seen the movie based on the true story, you must gift yourself by doing at least one or the other. It is a true story based around the lives of a Wesleyan pastor and his family who were changed forever by their four-year-old's visit to heaven. Your belief about an afterlife will be surely strengthened.

A little known fact about me is that I was raised in the Wesleyan Church in Malone, New York, where my parents attended when their health would allow.

Out of the Womb

My own labor pains were something I could never have imagined, even after being a nurse for many years and attending to so many births. You just can't fathom it, right mothers?

As I recall my first labor experience of forty-eight plus hours, I believe the not-so-kind words I uttered in those last tumultuous hours were definitely related to my fear of what could happen to my newborn baby while he was attempting to leave his first *home*. It was time to get my point across that there was no way I could deliver Jimmy the normal way...and I was right!

Birth and death are very similar in that for a baby it is truly leaving the familiar, passing into the unknown. As so it is with the dying. But knowing where you anticipate going after death can put a whole different spin on how the dying reacts at that moment.

Welcome Home

Countless times I have heard my hospice patients say, "I want to go home." It sometimes becomes a guessing game for loved ones to figure out which home is desired. If the right questions are asked, it is soon discovered that my patients are referring to their heavenly home. I get such joy when I feel assured that heaven is where these dear ones anticipate going, soon to be stepping into God's dressing room.

Just days prior to my Uncle Bob's death, he would say to my Aunt Donnamae, "I want to go now. I want to go home." She believes, as I do, he was talking about his heavenly home.

When Dad was in the Potsdam Emergency Room, and without any medication yet administered, he had a vision. He was sitting on the end of his stretcher, his legs dangling down, as it was much easier for him to breathe upright. I sat slightly behind him off the stretcher side and he leaned his back against me for support.

Dad calmly asked, "Judy, do you see that little boy standing in the corner?"

"No, Dad, I don't. How old do you think he is, and do you recognize him?"

"Oh, probably five or so. No, I don't know him."

"That's so nice of him to be here for you, Dad."

'Yes, yes, it is."

But that wasn't his last vision. After he was discharged home on comfort care/hospice care, he was in the hospital bed in the living room, sitting in an upright position. He asked, "Do you see that boy in the corner?"

"No, Dad, I don't. Do you know him?"

"No, I don't."

Neither of these visions frightened Dad but brought him comfort. It opened a conversation for us to have about visions experienced by so many, living and dying. Just days before Dad's death, his neighbor Roman was visiting. He asked Dad how he was doing, and Dad said, "I feel like I am between two different worlds."

With God's approval, we will be reunited with those who have stepped through the door ahead of us. We do not have to be a Mother Teresa, Billy Graham, or a Pope from Rome to get into heaven. We may have lived under a bridge with only the clothes on our back. Either way, the heavenly choir will be singing, Dad included, as Jesus welcomes us home. What an absolute joyous afterlife that will be.

3 Caring for the Dying

What do you think dying looks like, feels like, smells like, and sounds like? What are the greatest needs of the dying and how do you respond to each? How does one know when death is near?

Undoubtedly, all these questions and concerns will cross your mind if and when the time comes for you to be a caregiver for the dying. I am near certain that you will accomplish greater things than you ever dreamed capable of and that providing end-of-life care will change you, hopefully for the better.

Even the thought of being a caregiver of the dying, or being the one who is dying, can cause anxiety, referred to as *death anxiety*. Yet the concerns of caregiving can often be anticipated and easily surmounted by learning as much as possible before your care giving is needed.

Three Daughters and their Mother

I want to begin with a very compassionate mother who I met during her daughter's end-of-life hours one steamy, hot Florida morning. This precious little mom was caring for her baby-boomer daughter who was dying of breast cancer. The very saddest part of the whole story is this was her third daughter she cared for who would succumb to this illness.

After I took care of my patient's needs, her mother silently escorted me back to her front door. There she threw her arms around me, collapsed in my arms, and sobbed uncontrollably.

"I am so sorry, so very sorry," I said repeatedly as I cradled her in my arms the best I could.

What words could I ever speak to ease the emotional pain and heaviness of heart she was burdened with? As a mother myself, I knew she has had years of joy in her life with her three daughters, yet my mind couldn't imagine the severity of her sorrow.

I found myself angry with God as I stomped my way back to my van. I demanded an answer from Him: *Why in the world, Lord, did this happen to this mother? Why was she chosen to endure all this sadness in her middle and later years? Will her son be able to care for her like her daughters could have? Can someone please explain this to me before I throw in my towel of hospice nursing?* This visit was one of the most heart-wrenching ones in all my years of nursing.

Then it came to me! I realized that these three sisters will be so excited when they are hopefully reunited in heaven after being apart for so many years! Then can you imagine their renewed excitement and joy when their mom arrives, the one who lovingly cared for each one of them? There will be no more suffering or sorrow for any of those women, just pure joy!

Lie in my bed

Imagine yourself dressed in a hospital gown, lying in a hospital bed covered with colorless sheets, side rails enclosed around you, barren walls glaring back at you, and fluorescent lights staring down upon you.

There is a side table just out of your reach, heavily burdened with a bottle of generic lotion, an emesis basin, several mouth swabs, a plastic cup, a water pitcher and a meal tray with foul-smelling pureed foods begging to be touched.

Attached to one side rail is your only connection to the outer walls, a bell to push with the hopes of a timely response before your bladder spills over or your pain returns.

On the wall at the foot of your bed hangs a dry erase board with unfamiliar names to whom your care has been entrusted *yesterday*.

Hanging precariously from the ceiling is a television that drones news that depresses the healthy and certainly the ill.

Outside the door, you hear the alarming of machines begging for attention, frequent clanging noises from an assortment of delivery carts and stretchers, and call bells ringing and ringing and ringing.

Your most urgent thought and plea to your physician, who informed you that you may have only a short time to live, is, "Can I please go home to die?"

You have appreciated the care that you have received in the hospital but now home is where you want to be, where you want to die. How can that be?

Less than twenty-four hours later, your wish has been granted and you are home under the care of hospice. So now what happens? A whole new and positive outlook on truly living your final days has emerged with the expertise of a professionally trained and choreographed hospice team to assist you.

Despite the news of your approaching death, your terminal illness you were confronted with in the hospital can look, feel, smell, and sound completely different in your beloved home.

So Dad's story continues…

My dad and I talked frequently on the phone because we were 1,350 miles apart for most of my adult life. The one phone call I recall the most occurred in April 2022. I, of course, did not know he would be with Jesus within a month of that call. But my Dad knew. He said, "You need to come home." I asked, "What's the matter, Dad?" He responded, "I am not doing too well."

If you ever asked my dad how he was doing, he would inevitably say, "Pretty good." This time he said, "My chest pain is getting much worse, it goes from the front right through my back, and it hurts to breathe. My pain pill is not helping. Can you come soon?"

My husband's and my trip north had already been planned within a week of Dad's request as my sister and her family were going to Florida on vacation. So without hesitation we packed our car and our dog Jake and headed north earlier than planned.

When we walked into the living room and saw Dad, it was obvious he was in much distress, and very possibly approaching the end of his life. I assessed his vital signs, checked for swelling in his feet, and asked him detailed questions. He refused to go to the emergency room then but the next day he asked me to take him.

The ER doctor explained to Dad how very ill he was and must stay in the hospital for 2-3 days of treatment if he had any chance of surviving, or then he may not. Well, I will only add that he did return home the next day and was sent back to emergency rooms twice more in less than a month, including a transfer to Burlington Vermont Hospital, and the last one to Potsdam Hospital.

While in the Potsdam Emergency Room, two doctors cared for Dad who carefully examined him and questioned him about his symptoms. Countless blood tests were done, EKG, and a Cat Scan over several hours. Then one of the doctors entered the room and sat squarely in front of Dad, while I stood behind Dad.

The doctor asked a synopsis of questions I have heard doctors ask countless times to ensure their patient fully comprehends what is being said to them.

"Can you tell me your full name, please?

Dad did.

"Can you tell me your birthday?

Dad did.

"Can you tell me where you are?"

Dad did.

"Can you tell me what year it is?

Dad did.

"Can you tell me who is president?

Dad did.

"Mr. Fairchild, the other doctor that examined you and I have carefully reviewed your history, all your bloodwork, EKG, and your Cat Scan, plus your records from Burlington Hospital. You are a very sick man, especially due to your heart failing, plus the fluid is back around your lungs."

Dad knowingly shook his head yes.

The doctor paused then continued, "Plus... you have cancer in your blood."

Dad shook his head yes again, acknowledging his awareness of that.

The doctor continued, "We can send you to a large hospital to determine the type of your cancer, check your bone marrow, and determine options for treatment."

Dad shook his head no and whispered, "No, no, no, no". I spoke not a word.

The doctor offered to keep Dad several days to get his pain under control, plus his cough and shortness of breath. The doctor talked with Dad about comfort care, end of life care, care in his home for the terminally ill... called hospice care. He stressed that comfort meds would be available and medical equipment, including oxygen.

Without hesitation, and with Dad not asking for my opinion or any other family member, he said, "I want to go home with that." And so one of his final decisions in life was easily made by him and he made it without delay. Dad knew what was the absolute best and most comfortable option for him to "be with Shirl", my mother. So, after 2 nights in the Potsdam Hospital, and 6 days and 5 nights at home Dad died where he wanted, without pain, no coughing, no anxiety, and no shortness of breath, in peace with Mom sitting by his side, holding his hand, with her caregiver Tonyea kneeling by her and me comforting Dad as he stepped into heaven.

After Dad died, I was told he stated to some family members he never wanted to be on hospice. Yet when hospice care was explained to him by professionals and acknowledged his approaching death, Dad knew that was what he needed and wanted. And he knew I would be with him till the end. Thank you to the Hospice of the North Country in Malone for providing Dad with exceptional care, medications, and medical equipment; and to Mom's caregivers, Tonyea and Bernice, for sharing their knowledge of end-of-life care; Pastor Billy Bond; to Dad's neighbor and friend Shawn who helped care for Dad in all hours of the day and night. (Shawn, Dad loved you like a son.) And especially to my Aunt Donnamae who helped care for Dad, spent many days and nights when he was so ill, and has gifted so much to Dad and Mom.

Joy at the End-of-Life

When many people hear the word hospice, they think of death fast approaching, maybe even within just a few hours or a few days. In actuality, hospice care is available for those of all ages whose physician determines one's life expectancy is six months or less. *However,* dying is not that predictable and so patients may require hospice care for approximately a year or even more, care that is available twenty-four hours a day, seven days a week by a team of professionals.

One of my sweetest and most appreciative of patients (whose name was Joy) voiced her guilty feelings regarding her year-long need for hospice services. I would have visited Joy far longer than that if she had needed me to. She was one of my greatest teachers and caring for her while she battled cancer was a very humbling experience, never a job. In her memory, I have always included joy in the title of my end-of-life books.

Once medications are adjusted and symptoms are managed, a patient's condition may improve considerably while on hospice and may no longer be considered terminal. Then the physician, together with the patient, caregivers, and hospice staff, may decide hospice care is not needed and he/she will be discharged. Hospice care can be resumed when and if needed in the future.

When I discuss hospice care with those not familiar, the vast majority of them have thought that hospice is mainly for patients who have cancer, but that is not so. Approximately fifty percent of hospice patients have cancer and others have heart disease, kidney failure, Alzheimer's or Parkinson's disease, AIDS, lung disease, liver disease, general debility, Lou Gehrig's disease, Multiple Sclerosis, etc.

One of the main focuses of hospice is to improve one's quality of life by providing palliative care which addresses the control of symptoms for whatever the disease process may be.

As a hospice patient, you will be provided an interdisciplinary team of professionals who will address specific needs that you or your loving caregivers may have as you approach your death. Team members will visit you regularly and in emergency situations, addressing your physical, spiritual, emotional and psychosocial concerns and needs. Nurses, Social Workers, Chaplains, Home Health Aides and Certified Nursing Assistants, Volunteers, Complementary Therapists, Physical Therapists, Physicians, Bereavement Counselors, and countless support staff are available as part of hospice care.

While lying in your own bed, covered with linens the shade of plums, you no longer are wearing a hospital gown but pajamas familiar and comfortable, surrounded by your very attentive family, while your cat stretches out at the foot of your bed. Your bedroom walls are graced with a soothing honey color, and photos of smiling and loving faces look down upon you.

The person lying in your bed beside you is the one you have loved and cherished for many years, the one who knows your likes and dislikes, the one destined years ago to be your caregiver in sickness and in health and to forever love and to cherish.

If your physical needs require it and you so desire, hospice can provide home medical equipment that may give more comfort and allow ease in providing physical care for you. The same kind of hospital bed and side table that are in hospitals can be supplied in the home. Other potentially needed medical equipment may include a commode, oxygen, nebulizer for breathing treatments, wheelchair, walker, or cane.

Another benefit to hospice patients is the medications their doctor orders that *relate to their terminal illness* can be provided through hospice, which may result in a significant financial savings. Each patient often has their own doctor who orders the medications needed and follows the patient while receiving hospice care. A specialty trained hospice doctor may be available and may be requested to provide care, also.

Lou Gehrig's Disease

You will have to look long and very, very hard to find a wife, mother, grandmother, artist, and hospice nurse that will fill the shoes of Mary Freeman. I know because I worked with Mary for more than a dozen years. I am honored that she chose to share her family's very powerful and intimate story with you:

It was late in February, a chilly, sunny, busy day. My husband, Charlie, had been sick with Lou Gehrig's Disease for five years. He had been doing very poorly the previous month, and the kids, understanding my dread, had been hovering around as close as they could.

The kids- my salvation, comfort, support system, amusement, annoyance. They were additionally my helpers, sick-husband caretakers, frontline responders, and lifesavers. They were very young when he was diagnosed and very young when he died. They learned how a ventilator works and how to handle an ambu bag. The older two children knew how to set up and do tracheostomy suction, as well as routine care. They waited up until he was transferred into bed from his chair each night. They could all manage tube feedings. They all knew the drill for power failure, hurricanes, and broken or nonfunctioning equipment.

Yet, they did homework and watched TV, had friends over, and remained in his line of vision. When he couldn't move or smile or speak, they stayed with him, talked to him, and continued to have lives that included him every waking minute. My oldest daughter would ask me to leave the room so she could speak with him privately.

The day he died- the sunny, busy, seemingly ordinary day started as usual. Everyone went off to school…I got my husband bathed, dressed, and out of bed and into his chair. He had changed; he was lethargic and pale. Every instinct told me that he had started to die. I called his dearest friend, who was also his physician. He offered hospital admission, tests, IVs, and medical support. After five years of a really tough struggle, I thought that the time had come to say loving goodbyes and let him go.

When the kids came home from school, I explained that Daddy was dying and that they could stay in the house or in the room, or they could go home with a very beloved friend and wait with her, and that this was very peaceful for him, and the end of a very long journey. They all stayed. They said their goodbyes with hugs and tears and waited outside the room. My husband's mother came, as well as all the "in-town" relatives. Our dearest friends came and went.

At the end, there were three of us with him: his buddy the doctor, my buddy an oncology nurse, and me. It was a death where the light gets dimmer and dimmer, the heart rate slower and slower, and the moment of death is indistinct. They waited for me to turn off the ventilator- and they also let me get the kids. We all visited with him until I called the funeral director. I sent the kids out so I could wash him and get him ready. My second child, little Charlie, then twelve–years-old, wanted to help... and so we did it together.

When a funeral director arrives, they usually request that family members leave the room. But Charlie said to the funeral director that he had been taking care of his father all along, and he would do this last thing for him. So he helped to wrap him up, move him to the stretcher, and put him all the way into the van. He only stepped back when the doors were closed, and he held my hand until the van was gone.

My husband loved kids and all the friends of my children came back to the house after the funeral. At nightfall, all bundled up in the cold, we all went to the dock behind our house and set off firecrackers and told stories about him. It is a good memory to keep.

Who will be with you when you die?

Who do you want with you when you are dying? Many of us have never given it a thought nor realized the significance in choosing our caregiver at the end of our life. Do you realize how important it is for that certain someone (or two or three) to know they are the chosen ones to be at your bedside?

Family and close friends become a critical component for the dying, especially if they wish to die at home. I have seen adult sons and daughters tenderly care for their mothers and fathers. But I have also seen close friends and neighbors, grandchildren, stepchildren, church members, nieces and nephews, in-laws and perhaps, unknown to me, outlaws providing care. The chosen ones are sometimes those you would least expect.

When it comes to the bedside of the dying, you can spot a best friend from the doorway or over the phone lines. She or he may be a neighbor, a classmate, a co-worker, a sister or brother, an aunt or mother, a spouse… someone who is willing to lovingly care for you at the end of your life, knowing there is no way the favor can ever be returned.

What care giving is really all about is who is at your bedside *willingly*, who has the privilege of being there, for that is truly what it is.

I Choose you

I received an email several years ago that said God would send us carefully chosen friends depending on what we needed at the time. For example, if you are having a tough time with your teenager, He will send you a friend who also has a teenager and understands what troubles you are having and can provide you with support.

If your car breaks down in the wee hours of the morning, it may be just minutes from a friend who has the ability to tow you home.

Perhaps your mother has taken ill and you are concerned about a new medication she is taking so you call your friend who is a pharmacist. Bingo! You are a recipient of God's chosen friend.

You may not truly discover who your best friends, loved ones, or closest family members are until you are lying on your deathbed. They are the ones who compassionately provide intimate care when needed, be a sincere spokesperson when the dying is unable, and sit vigil as death approaches. These exceptional caregivers want to learn as much as they can about death and dying so they can provide the best of care to a loved one or patient. Dad's neighbor/friend Shawn helped me so many times in Dad's last weeks, and Dad so appreciated him.

It touches me emotionally when I visit my hospice patients and there sits their best friend next to the bedside holding their hand, changing their clothing or linens on their bed, or cleaning the commode, helping them figure out what to eat that won't make them sicker, and then try to fix it if it does.

These best friends may be performing manicures or helping with a shower, gently placing their best friend in a wheelchair and taking them for a stroll outside, or rubbing their achy back with soothing lotion.

If times seem too tough to handle then your best friend may pray with you and ask for God's comfort and guidance in your hours of need.

Those caring for you may become your voice when you cannot be understood and a trustworthy advocate to speak on your behalf, whether it is to a doctor, nurse, lawyer, family member, landlord, etc.

Those are the chosen ones that won't expect or want anything in return.

In the Absence of a Caregiver

The challenges and responsibilities of raising a family and tending to their needs are of utmost importance but, no matter how much we wish we could temporarily walk away to care for someone else, sometimes it just cannot be done. It is important to recognize and accept that these situations or personal responsibilities take priority. Certainly, I would not expect someone with a child to forfeit his or her care for mine.

Social Workers can be a great resource for families who need guidance in choosing in-home care, private caregivers, or facility placement, if needed.

The Next Best Thing to Home

There are many homes away from home where those approaching death reside, short-term or long-term, and are able to receive hospice care there. In hospitals, nursing homes, assisted living facilities, private residential homes, shelters, or hospice care centers are all places end-of-life patients may reside.

You may have a Hospice Care Center or Hospice Home in your neighborhood, with 24/7 staff present, and not recognize it as such. It may appear to be a five star hotel or a welcoming home we are most familiar with. A Chapel and/or Memorial Garden may be available which can provide a place for private prayer and reflection.

Hospice centers are decorated in a home-like fashion but with all the necessities those approaching death may need. On the walls and on the dressers are displayed mementos and pictures of loved ones, exuding the feeling of home.

A Day in May

It was high noon at the end of May. The air was sticky and heavy each time I exited my car during my weekend visits, one of which included a stop at a nursing home to assess a lady I will call Mae.

Upon my arrival in Mae's room, she was lying in a hospital bed on her left side, her back to the door. Her daughter sat behind her mother at the edge of her bed.

After I introduced myself, I walked around the foot of the bed to Mae's left side and, while leaning over her side rail, I said, "Mae, I'm Judy, your visiting nurse. I'm here to see how you're doing today." As I gently laid my hand on her head, she opened her eyes and looked directly at me for a very brief moment. I asked her daughter if she'd like to sit at her mother's left side so when she opened her eyes again so she would see her there. The daughter declined, stating that she was okay where she was.

As I assessed this feeble little lady, her daughter explained the circumstances that occurred during the night and how her family had gathered vigil at her bedside, singing hymns and praying together.

Because I felt Mae's death may occur within a day or two, it was important to leave her bedside for a few minutes so I could explain to her daughter in private the events that may occur. After telling my patient that we would be back in a few minutes, we convened outside her room. At this time, Mae showed no signs that she was just minutes from dying.

Her daughter and I discussed what changes are often exhibited in someone prior to death and, even though this daughter was very tearful, she knew her mother was ready to enter heaven. The family had discussed it openly with Mae before her stroke and all were aware of her imminency.

As we returned to the bedside, her daughter and I noticed very apparent changes in her mother's condition. Her breathing had become very irregular and I believed she was within minutes of dying. Her daughter immediately called her younger sister, requesting she come as soon as possible.

I lowered the rails on the bed so my patient's adult child could sit on the edge of the bed next to her. Mae's eyes remained closed, with her head now rigidly turned to the left, away from her daughter. She was not responsive at all to our voice or touch. Her hands and feet were cool with diminished circulation, and her skin had a bluish hue.

As we waited together, Mae's daughter started singing and praying for her mother and spoke sweetly to her about heaven and how everyone who had gone before her, including Jesus, were waiting for her. Mae's breathing became even slower. Her daughter continued pouring out her love for her mother, and then she started singing a very old hymn I knew: "I've got a mansion just over the hilltop…" so I quietly joined her in song.

Nearly twenty minutes had passed since our return to Mae's side. Then very unexpectedly, Mae turned her previously rigid head fully from her left side to her right side and stared at her little girl with wide open and unflinching eyes. At that moment, I felt a tingling sensation cover one side of my body; I knew the angels were present. Mae then turned her head back to where she'd been facing prior. Just then her second daughter entered the room, and Mae took her last breath.

I have never felt a spirit as strong around me as Mae's was. She surely must have been a very special lady and I was blessed to have been with her upon her entry into heaven.

A Teardrop

Lacy and I had been neighbors for many years. She was a businesswoman and, without a doubt, a beautiful lady. Unfortunately, Lacy had been diagnosed with Alzheimer's disease and her life would change drastically.

Because our Florida weather is typically very mild and warm, most of the neighborhood folks spend a lot of time outside. Neither Lacy nor I were any different. So when I saw Lacy out of her house I would wave to her and say, "Hi, Lacy!" With that simple acknowledgment, Lacy would either turn and shuffle back into her home or hide behind a corner and peer around at me. She would not speak to me, as her illness would not allow her to.

Lacy's health declined rather quickly, but I continued to reach out to her in my simple way. She showed no sign of emotion or willingness to communicate with me, yet I often wondered if she recognized my attempt to reach her.

When Lacy became bedridden, I went to see her in her home as she was now receiving hospice care. As I approached Lacy, she stared very intently at me. I thought my heart would explode as it pounded in my chest because I did not want to upset Lacy in her last days on earth, but I so much wanted to be with her and support her husband, as well. I wanted to somehow try to ease her fear and let her know I was not there to hurt her.

As with nearly all my other visits, I found myself kneeling next to Lacy's bedside to be eye level with her. I didn't touch my friend, as I didn't want to frighten her by invading her personal space. I hesitated to speak but finally said the standard greeting I used across the lawn a thousand times, "Hi, Lacy."

Lacy's face remained stoic, as it had been for so many months. Her eyes were set deep into her face. She didn't blink or frown. She looked straight at me with a very peaceful look on her face. Then slowly, from out of the corner of her eyes, Lacy shed tears, silent tears.

I believe that Lacy's look of peace and the shedding of her tears was the only way she could communicate that she had known each time I spoke to her, when I tried to reach out to her, when I tried to help her, when I tried to console her, when I tried to fix her shoe, help her with her car door, or acknowledge how pretty she looked on any particular day. I thanked God for showing me the understanding that had always been tucked inside Lacy's soul. How happy I was that she would soon be set free from her disease.

Ethel's Back

Lawrence's wife, Ethel, had died seven months prior to my visit with Lawrence and his family. They all spoke so highly of Ethel and missed her dearly.

Unfortunately, shortly after Ethel's death, Lawrence noticed some difficulty breathing, especially with any exertion or exercise. Plus, he had a nagging cough. So off to the doctor Lawrence went, only to find out that he had lung cancer which was far beyond any successful chance of treatment.

During my visit, I sat together with the family in the sun-filled living room where we discussed what lay ahead for their father and them. As we talked, the family shared stories of their dad and recent events involving their mother. They said that one day Lawrence was sitting in his recliner with his feet up when he jumped as if startled by something. Lawrence said, "Ethel, be more careful now! You just brushed against my feet!" Lawrence was certain Ethel was present and reminding him she was patiently waiting for him.

The Comfort of Pets

Pets have a great sense as to when their loved one is approaching death, often displayed by their increased attentiveness and/or protectiveness of their master. Several stories reveal the power of pets.

After ringing the doorbell of my patient Julie's home, I was greeted by her husband who welcomed me in and directed me to his wife. It was difficult to see Julie nestled in the corner of her couch in the darkened living room as the shades were all drawn.

I was quite startled when the quiet house suddenly filled with the defensive barking of a terrier dog named Sparky. His four little feet were swiftly planted squarely in front of mine, blocking my approach to Julie. The loving master of Sparky reassured me that he wouldn't bite but only barks a lot in an effort to claim the center of attention and protect his territory and family.

After stepping across the shiny tile floor, with Sparky at my heels, I sat next to Julie on her sofa made of a beautiful fabric of paisley roses in tweed. I first noticed her abdomen was very distended, which caused her to rest back deep into the couch, allowing her more room to breathe. The scowl on her pale face portrayed a look of discomfort and discontent. My new cancer patient's symptoms were based on the fact that her routine medicine was not effectively easing her nausea as it had in the past. So after reviewing what she had available in her home, I placed a call to the hospice triage nurse, who would contact Julie's doctor and give him an update on her condition and medication needs.

After addressing other concerns and clarifying medication changes, the topic turned to something that Julie said had been weighing heavily on her mind for days.

"Judy, please tell me what is going to happen to me and my body when I get closer to dying," she pleaded.

I took a slow, deep breath and mentally asked the heavens above to guide me in using the right words, as I knew Julie wanted me to be very open and honest with her. Together, hand in hand, I told this beautiful new friend of mine what to expect, reassuring her that she will most likely have a very peaceful death as she slips further into a deep sleep.

Julie and I talked about how her hopes of beating her cancer would now focus more on her hope for a peaceful and pain-free death, with her family and close friends surrounding her and comforting each other until she died. We spoke of angels that would gather around her and the likelihood that this faith-filled woman sitting next to me may also have visions of heaven and of loved ones already passed. Her parents were very dear to Julie, and she said she missed them terribly since their deaths and wanted to be with them again soon.

As the sun peeked slightly around the living room shades, she voiced a comfort and relief in knowing what may occur in the future. She stated she was no longer afraid since she had confronted her fear of dying, proving to herself that her courage and love of family and friends would sustain her in her final days, hours, and minutes.

After tearful hugs and sweet goodbyes, I left a very weak, middle-aged lady still sitting in the corner of her favorite couch. I then walked back across the tile with the fuzzy little terrier yipping behind me all the way. After turning to say goodbye, my new patient and friend raised her hand and said, "Thank you for helping me in so many ways!"

Several months passed before I was called back to Julie's house. After entering the same front door, I noticed the empty couch in the living room where she and I had sat before. The shades were still drawn, but there was no barking Sparky. I entered the bedroom in the back of her home and at the foot of Julie's bed lay a silent Sparky. The little terrier turned and looked at me but did not utter a sound.

Julie was lying on her left side, her eyes closed, and her expression peaceful. A spray of light from a golden sunset shone through her bedroom window onto the foot of her bed. I kneeled on the floor at her side, placing myself at eye level with her. I gently placed her right hand in mine and softly spoke her name.

"Julie." Pause. "Julie."

Julie opened her beautiful green eyes slightly and looked squarely into mine for a brief moment. She moved her lips but was too weak to speak, so I slowly spoke to her. "This is Judy, your hospice nurse. I am here to see you again. I know you are very, very weak, and it is difficult to speak."

Julie's lips moved, but no sound came out. Through tiny little slits in her eyes, she continued to look squarely into mine.

"I am here to help you. Is that ok?"

Julie slowly blinked twice.

I gently continued, "Julie, I know you remember our talk several months ago. We talked about dying, and I believe you are near to dying. Do you feel that way?"

The pale eyelids blinked twice, and together our eyes misted up.

"Your husband told me all of your family are coming back to see you tonight, so they will be here to help and comfort you, too."

Julie slowly closed her eyes.

I paused for nearly a minute before proceeding. "Julie, do you remember me telling you that angels would gather around your bed before you die?"

Suddenly, this angelic lady, who was lying nearly motionless, had the most radiant smile I had ever seen! I was stunned, in awe, and humbled to be in such a holy place. There was no doubt in my mind that Julie sensed angels around her and knew they were preparing to take her to heaven very soon. How grateful I was.

After providing personal care and repositioning Julie under her down filled comforter, I bent down and gave her a kiss goodbye on her forehead and a very gentle hug. I thanked her for allowing me to share in this very intimate and sacred time in her life. Her final goodbye to me was a slight whisper from her lips, "Thank you, Judy."

Then my thoughts turned to Sparky. He knew what was happening as he never left Julie's side. He never once challenged my presence or caregiving, nor when her very tearful husband tended to her lovingly.

Many of my patients had a very special pet with an immense sense of its owner's approaching death. Some will not leave their side, except to *water* the lawn outside. Others become extremely protective, and it may be nearly impossible to safely approach their master. Family members frequently ask me what my opinion is as to whether their pets will one day join them in heaven. I leave my understanding to a certain translation from Ecclesiastes 3:18-21:

I also thought about the human condition— how God proves to people that they are like animals. For people and animals share the same fate— both breathe and both must die. So people have no real advantage over the animals. Both go to the same place— they came from dust and they return to dust. For who can prove that the human spirit goes up and the spirit of animals goes down into the earth?

Whether Sparky joins Julie one day in heaven or my Spooky joins me, I can only hope it will be. I do know that before the sun rose in the morning, the angels were singing *hallelujah* for Julie as she and her heavenly family had been reunited, just as she had predicted.

Arnie and Booter

Anne Buell Bashista, a co-worker of mine, witnessed first-hand the power of pets while caring for her husband, Arnie, who was diagnosed with pancreatic cancer.

Anne said Arnie's philosophy was "what will be, will be." He knew that he was going to die but he also was determined to live while he could.

Anne had spent months trying to talk Arnie into letting her get a cat and so when he finally relented Anne headed off to the animal shelter, returning home with her cat named Booter. However, it was Arnie and Booter that bonded like glue.

Every afternoon they would take their nap together- Arnie would sit in his recliner and Booter would get on his lap, lay across his knees, look up at him, put his right paw out, and Arnie would put his hand over it.

In February, Arnie started getting some back pain. X-rays showed that he had some metastasis in his lungs. He started losing weight and his energy level started decreasing. Annie said, "By summer, Arnie was losing weight so fast we couldn't keep him in anything that fit him. He would look at himself in the mirror and ask, 'Where did I go?' "

Anne says he still continued to be a positive person. He would say, "Just because I am sick doesn't mean that our lives are done!"

By October, Arnie consented to hospice care. He was having respiratory distress and was weaker, but still alert and oriented. Arnie told Anne, "Honey, don't take this the wrong way, but I just want it over. I'm so tired. You just can't know how it feels. It's time."

Anne told him that she understood and it was all right for him to go.

When nurses were present in the home during Arnie's final days, Booter kept a very strict eye on them, as he lay up on the hospital bed with Arnie. If Booter couldn't see Arnie, he would get up, turn around and lay back down again. He was very intense and very upset.

Anne continues her story, "Saturday morning Arnie kicked me out of the house for a couple of hours. The nurse told me when I got back that he had talked to his sons and said good-bye to them. He talked to my father and told him they were just doing some medication adjustments. He didn't want him to worry.

"Through Sunday, he just laid there with his eyes closed. He laughed once at something I said (for the life of me, I wish I could remember what it was)."

On Sunday, the hospice chaplain had been requested by Anne and arrived at 3:15pm. Arnie "raised his eyebrows up but still didn't open his eyes. Again his breathing changed."

Anne continues, "At 3:30pm, he seemed to still be very aware but was changing very rapidly.

"About twenty minutes later, he started moving around in the bed, lifted his upper body, moved closer to my side of the bed and said, 'Honey.' With him moving closer to me on the bed I really believe that he was saying his good-bye. It was only a couple of minutes later that he was gone.

"Booter was in the Florida room when Arnie died and they tell me he let out a scream and took off running. Later, when things were quiet, Booter got up on the bed and just sat there watching Arnie for a while. Finally, he went over to him and smelled at his mouth, gave him a kiss, a love bump on his forehead, and then went over the head of the bed. Booter had said good-bye to his dad. Arnie was a wonderful person and I miss him."

A Holy Coincidence

When I worked for hospice during the weekend, my patients would require symptom management, caregivers would need support or education in how to best care for their loved one, or a visit would be needed upon one's death. Generally, to begin my work day, unless there was an emergency, I would connect the hospice laptop computer I carried with me to the main computer so I am assured of the most up-to-date information on my patients.

On this one particular Sunday morning, for some unexplainable glitch, I was not able to send or receive the information I needed so it was decided that I would have to leave my laptop behind in the hospice office to be fixed so I could get to my patients in a timely fashion.

The day transpired into what I call a *holy coincidence,* as a higher power than I had to be at the helm.

After receiving a verbal report on my initial assignments of three patients and acquiring the medical supplies I anticipated needing, I headed to my van earlier than expected to begin my day. My initial patient needed a fasting blood sample drawn so I would go there first before she would eat her breakfast. However, just as I was preparing to leave the parking lot, the hospice triage nurse Diane phoned me from the office and said the patient called, wanted to eat breakfast *now*, and would not wait for my arrival. The patient chose to have the blood work completed the next day instead. So I was to continue on to my next patient.

My second patient, who had just been admitted to hospice the day prior, was twenty-five miles away so I arrived at his home approximately thirty minutes later.

After assessing my patient, providing some personal care and education, and clarifying his medication needs with him and his caregivers, I proceeded to my third patient who was only a few miles down the road.

As I approached my next patient's home, the front yard was very welcoming with colorful flowers along the tidy stone walkway leading me to the front door. Just several feet inside the home lay my patient in a hospital bed. This gentle man greeted me with a cheery hello and immediately voiced his gratefulness for returning home the day prior after many days in the hospital. His wife reported he was doing much better than she had expected after his severe illness and was so relieved.

My patient's wife reported that an hour prior to my arrival, he had combed his hair, washed his own face, and was thoroughly enjoying his time at home with his adored wife, his son, daughter-in-law, and granddaughter who had just recently arrived from out of state, plus his very beloved little dog. After their dog yipped at me for several minutes, he recognized I wasn't a threat to his ailing master so he settled and accepted my presence.

Together the family spoke of their life together, their love for the Lord, and how they missed attending their local church where many of their longtime friends were at this very hour. His wife expressed her thankfulness that their pastor visited the day prior and they expected church members to stop in and visit after the service was completed this morning.

The next twenty minutes I remember very clearly.

The main purpose of my visit was to redress a simple surgical wound for this gentle man. After assessing his vital signs and gathering my medical supplies, I began with his dressing change. I noticed the time we began was 11:00 a.m. just as their church service would have begun.

During the next ten minutes, his daughter-in-law, who is also a nurse, assisted me as I redressed his wound and straightened his linens. Just as I was completing his care, this gentleman's breathing began to change. He developed a wet juicy sound in the back of his throat and could speak only a few words at a time due to his shortness of breath. He was very calm and had no fear or pain exhibited on his face or with his body language. He very clearly asked, "Can I go now?" His wife thought maybe he wanted to get up in his chair and she assured him that he could when I was done. I very soon realized he was talking about going to heaven, as many of our patients imply as going to as death nears.

The ache in the pit of my stomach and my years caring for the dying heightened my awareness that my patient was probably and almost unbelievably just minutes from dying. His daughter-in-law had also recognized his very rapid decline and stayed close to her mother-in-law, who now also noticed a major change in her husband's condition. I gently and lovingly comforted my patient, his wife and family. I quietly explained to his wife what I thought was occurring as I noticed his color was becoming paler and he was becoming unresponsive to voice or touch. His breathing had become quieter and slower.

His wife wrapped her arms gently around him and repeatedly said, "I love you, I love you." The little dog was carried to the bedside and was abnormally quiet and somewhat shaky, as he attended to his loving owner.

Twenty minutes after eleven, forty minutes after my arrival, this loving man took his last, peaceful breath on earth.

The only words that made much sense at that moment were that this man of faith entered heaven when his church friends and pastor would have been in prayer, certainly praying for one of their own.

If my computer had not malfunctioned, if my first patient had not cancelled her visit, and if my second patient had been further from my last, I would not have been witness to such a *holy coincidence*. God puts us where we are supposed to be.

Time to Huddle and Cuddle

As I whispered my greeting to my patient Angela, I anticipated no response from her as I thought she was in a deep sleep or coma. However, my lack of faith in her was quickly dispelled when she snapped open her eyes and, with a cheery grin, said "Hello. And who are you?"

That was an easy enough question for me to answer. Then as Angela smiled even broader, followed by a twinkle in her deep set brown eyes, I concluded this would be one of my most memorable visits.

Before I could respond to Angela, she continued, "So, what are you here for?"

Her daughter spoke up and said, "Actually, Mom, I asked a nurse to come."

"What for? I don't need anything."

It can be a very touchy situation when a visit from a hospice team member is requested without the patient's permission, especially when the patient is capable of making those decisions. However, when approached correctly, it nearly always turns out to be a benefit for the patient and the caller.

"Just to make sure you don't need anything and that we are doing the right thing," her daughter added, as her brothers stood a distance from the hospital bed.

The previously vague reason for my visit soon unfolded as a conversation of dying, visions of angels, and heaven began. There was no look of fear or anxiety related to dying on Angela's face. However, several of her children exhibited just that. One son stood in the farthest corner of his mom's room, while the others gathered intermittently close by, occasionally taking their mom's hand and sharing in the heavenly conversation about what life would be like in the hereafter.

As my visit progressed, each of her devoted children became more comfortable holding her hand, touching her face, and expressing a desire to be closer physically to her. So the bed railings were lowered, and each of the children sat next to her or crawled up alongside of her, wrapping their arms around her and holding her gently as she had held them for many tender years. With a new understanding of death as being gentle and filled with a peace that passes all understanding, each felt comfortable in being close to their mother, sharing words they were once hesitant to say, and not afraid to show affection for their mother as they did when they were children.

When I leave the bedside of a patient like Angela, I never know when they will die. But if I recognize that death is imminent, the importance of being open and honest about their approaching death is paramount to my visits.

The days and hours Angela had left with her children would provide the much needed closure between them all. Together, their love and faith would sustain them through the dying process and rebirth to heaven, which occurred one week from the day of our visit.

There have been homes I have visited where I was instructed before stepping across the threshold of the front door that I am not to mention death, dying, hospice, or any other word that may cause the patient to construe that he or she is dying. In fact, I have had to remove my name badge so no sign of hospice was visible. But we must honor the wishes of those involved and can only hope that the acceptance of one's approaching death is more imminent than death itself.

A Visit from Grandpa

Grandparents around the world have protected their grandbabies as long as time has been recorded. Grandparents have been deemed by some as the forgotten grievers and perhaps grandchildren, also.

My twenty-three-year-old hospice patient shared in her grief, her love, and her loneliness for her deceased grandfather. She told me how he always understood her so well and so she wasn't surprised it was her grandfather that saved her day, years after his death. She explained, "I told my husband through my tears that I cannot do it anymore. No more chemotherapy." Her latest treatments made her so sick that she told her husband it was impossible for her to have any quality of life any longer and the treatments were to stop.

Later that day, when alone and sobbing into her pillow, she sensed someone in the room with her. As she lifted her head from out of her pillow she saw her grandfather standing at the foot of her bed. Without any words spoken, she said he gently placed his hands on her feet which immediately initiated a very warm sensation that moved up her entire body. Miraculously, within twenty minutes her symptoms totally subsided and she was able to get out of bed and attend to her child and husband, which she hadn't been able to do for some time.

Grandpa Fairchild

While in nursing school, I had the honor to practice my new care giving skills on a well-loved patient, my Grandfather Vincent. He resided in a nursing home and on occasion, when he was able, he would go to his home for several hours on a weekend. If I was home from college, I would go and help transfer Grandpa from his wheelchair to his bed, so he could take a short nap, and then back to his wheelchair. It was a tricky thing to do with me weighing in at 102 lbs. (which is definitely not what I weigh now) and Grandpa easily doubling my size. Believe it or not, there is a safe way for nearly everyone to transfer someone under these conditions. Allow me to regress a bit for the main gist of the story.

On the morning I left for my very first day of college devastating news struck the Fairchild family. My grandfather had a massive stroke and left him totally paralyzed on one side of his body, near mute, and understandably very depressed and withdrawn. He was nothing like the Grandpa I knew.

My Grandma's faith and belief in an all-powerful God gave her the assurance that the love of her life could be healed and so without a doubt she asked her church's pastor and the church's District Superintendent, who was also a pastor, to say prayers over Grandpa asking God to totally heal him from his severe disability.

Before the private prayer service, the minister spoke with my father Carlton, Grandma and Grandpa's second oldest son, and asked what he thought his mother's expectations were. My dad assured him that Grandma expected a total healing!

With that in mind, a private prayer service was held with Grandpa, Grandma, Dad, the local pastor, and the District Superintendent present.

A miracle did happen but not the one Grandma expected. Grandpa was not healed physically but rather he was healed spiritually and emotionally as after that prayer service he often smiled, held his head up, and joined in the camaraderie of his very large and extended family. He laughed sometimes with tears of joy as his belly shook like Jell-O, and he would join in conversation even though the only words he could speak were fewer than the fingers on his hands. He was grateful for every day of the ten years he lived thereafter with my Grandma visiting him nearly every day. Their six children all played an active role in his care giving. Of course, Grandpa had some down times just like we all do, but none would cause him deep depression like he had experienced before his miracle.

My father had never shared this story about Grandpa's private prayer service with anyone until over forty years after his healing. Dad was 89 then, seven years beyond the age my Grandpa was when he died.

What I learned from this story, and I sincerely hope you did, too, has been reinforced for multiple years through many of my patients and their families. There are different kinds of healing: physical, emotional, spiritual and mental, and we don't always get what we pray for… but sometimes what we get is far better than what we asked for.

A Constipated yet Jolly Soul

"I didn't know getting an enema could be a social event," my patient jokingly said. But that is exactly what it ended up being. So I termed a new word for the medical dictionary relating to just that- *celenemabration.*

When I initially explained to my new patient that what he needed was an enema, it truly became much more than that before we were through (I will spare you the intimate details). Throughout the procedure, my gentlest of gentlemen entertained me with the heartiest laugh and a belly full of cheer (and other predictable things) that could rouse anyone from the depths of despair, even if it entailed the assistance with bowel care. His wife shared his same good cheer and roared right along with us. Certainly, no one would have ever imagined that this man was in the midst of dying. He had many humorous stories to tell, but this one was most comical: "When I was in the hospital not long ago, a female nurse came into my room announcing that it was time for my bath. A bath? Hah! It ended up being more like a *car wash*! I had never experienced a bath like that! Then just as I was recovering from my car wash, a male nurse came into my hospital room. Through our conversation I shared with him my previous bathing adventure."

The belly laughs started again when my patient revealed that the male nurse joyously explained that the nurse who gave him his *car wash* was his wife! Oh how I loved the way my patient strived to create happiness in his home, and just because he needed to prepare for his death did not mean he had to stop enjoying life.

An Unexpected Translation

There are some condominiums on the east coast of Florida that require you to walk outside on their balconies or walkways to get to the front door. Of course, these doors my patients lie behind can be dozens of floors above the pavement below. That is not always a welcome thing especially if there is a strong and cold winter wind coming off the ocean, which causes my already frightful knees to rattle even more when at great heights.

Nonetheless, my hospice visit on this particular day was to assist the caregivers and my patient, who were a handful of flights above the pavement yet worth the hike up the stairs. Lilly's adult children were so relieved when I stepped through their doorway as they felt their mother was very close to dying and was uncertain as to what to expect and what to do. They told me their mother's native language was Spanish, which I know none, so I apologized for my lack of ability in communicating with her. They assured me that was not a concern at all. Another great story evolved.

After spending half her life in South America where she was born, Lilly moved to the United States. She spoke Spanish in her everyday household and learned just enough English so she could communicate some with those in her adopted country.

As Lilly approached dying, she became weaker and unfortunately took a tumble one day, injuring her hip. With no reasonable explanation, Lilly's preferred language suddenly changed from her native Spanish to speaking fluent English. As a result, what I thought would be a challenge in communicating with my hospice patient was not a challenge at all, for which her caregivers were very grateful for and me, too.

Long Time Coming

After I rang the doorbell of a previously visited home, the front door inched slightly open. The partial outline of a man's face peeking through the crack was barely visible, but it recalled memories of my earlier visit. After reassuring this elderly man that I had been to see him and his wife several months ago and was there to provide care for his wife again, he quickly opened the door. I was more surprised to see him nearly six months later than he was to see me. Because his wife was very ill during my last visit, I had expected her to die soon after.

After receiving a brief report on his wife's condition, Ted escorted me down a narrow hallway to their bedroom toward the back of their home. As I followed him, it was easy to see that perhaps Ted could also use some care as he slowly shuffled his feet across the barren floor, his shoulders stooped over from perhaps not only his ninety-one years but also from the weight of his months of care giving. When glancing around Ted, I saw the back of a wheelchair with a white-haired lady sitting in it. Her body was tilted slightly to the left, toward the side that was paralyzed. As I approached her right side she glanced sideways at me and boldly grumbled, "What took you so long?"

The circumstance surrounding my visit was related to Mrs. Ted falling off a chair earlier in the day. Fortunately, her husband was beside her and eased her to the floor so she suffered only a bruise to her right elbow. Ted was nearly in tears as he confessed that his wife's care had become too difficult for him due to her increased weakness. She was having great difficulty eating due to paralysis in her face, plus she was sleeping at very short intervals. Ted was exhausted mentally and physically.

So the circle of three, a beloved husband and wife and myself, had a long discussion about the need for more help provided by hospice staff to help ease the tremendous burden of care giving that Ted was responsible for. Unfortunately, they had no children and no family to help.

After assisting with Mrs. Ted's meal of chicken soup and then returning her to bed and giving her some medicine to relax her as they requested, I spoke privately with Ted. He knew that his wife was very close to dying this time, and he cried with all the strength he had left.

After hugs and reassurance that someone would be visiting them both again within just a few hours, he relaxed and was relieved to see that his wife was finally asleep.

I hardly ever know what happens once I leave a patient's home, since I only visit when a crisis or special need arises. However, I did learn that Mrs. Ted died within twelve hours of my leaving her bedside with her husband and another hospice nurse present. I did not expect her to die that quickly, but I knew she had been waiting at least six months for that moment... and she was ready. My thoughts turned to Ted in his loneliness, as he and his wife had been married for sixty-two years.

It may seem indifferent to some, but I am filled with a sense of peace when I discover that two loves such as these have been reconnected after their deaths.

A Child Near Death

A man introduced to me through a hospice co-worker was in my home servicing a piece of equipment. While working, he told me this story about his childhood miracle.

At near eighteen-months-old and able only to speak a few words, he was deathly ill with spinal meningitis. In fact, his doctor told his family that only a few days would lapse before their son's death. The family called their priest to the bedside to administer the last rites, baptize him, and give him communion. Certainly, no one expected him to recognize or remember anything that occurred around him due to his young age and his grave condition, if he survived.

To the amazement and gratefulness of everyone, in the few days that followed, he awoke. What increased everyone's amazement even more was that this toddler began speaking in full sentences, even recalling in detail some of the events that had occurred as he lay dying.

When he became a teenager, he felt the need to clarify what really happened to him as a very young child as it was never openly discussed in his presence all those years. After telling his mother and grandmother what he recalled, they both confirmed that what he had heard snippets of and felt certain occurred years prior was very true.

You are my Sunshine

Certain songs bring back lots of memories. Some songs recall happier times than others. I would bet that you could hum a tune now that holds a lot of meaning for you.

One of my songs is "You are my Sunshine." That is the song I have sung to my grandchildren since their births, and they can now sing-a-long with me.

On a Wednesday evening while visiting a patient new to hospice, we were having a great time conversing on all sorts of topics while addressing his health needs. Actually, I had just given him an enema and he felt so much better afterwards (yes, constipation is common).

I try to never miss an opportunity, when I feel it is appropriate, to put a smile on my patient and caregiver's faces and an enema certainly wouldn't prevent my attempt on this occasion. So I told my very grateful patient that maybe this would be a perfect occasion to sing a happy song! And so he began singing, "You are my sunshine, my only sunshine..."

I don't have to tell you how totally surprised I was that he chose that particular song out of the millions he could have chosen...another *holy coincidence*. Of course, I shared with him that I sing that song to my grandchildren all the time. He just smiled. I was hoping that I would have the opportunity to visit him and his wife again soon. However, he died four days later. I was so thankful I got at least one chance to share in their sunshine.

My next visit wasn't so enjoyable and certainly singing was not appropriate but a hospice chaplain visit was. Daniel was in his 90's, his wife in her 80's. He was ready to die but she wasn't ready to release him. Her denial, anger, and bitterness would be reflected onto numerous caregivers and family who did realize that Daniel didn't have the stamina or health to endure much more.

I offered a chaplain in hopes that would bring them some comfort and closure but she adamantly refused, as that would "only make things worse."

Then she openly showed me why she may have felt so angry and bitter. With a near-silent whisper, so Dan wouldn't hear, she pointed a finger down toward the floor and said that's where she expected they would go. Then pointing upward she said, "I doubt if we will go there."

My Uncle Jay

My Uncle Jay could have invented the word survivor and the concept of living until dying as he battled cancer for many years. But thankfully, like my dad, he loved adventure and was still able to take his wife/Aunt Golda, my parents, Uncle Dale and Aunt Eunice, Uncle Jack and Aunt Erma on many trips. My cousin, Rene Fairchild Kavanaugh, shares her father's story.

"I was very lucky because the last ten years of my dad's life, when he was at his most relaxed, I got to spend all the time with him because I was home as well. There were times that my dad wanted to do this, or go here, and sometimes I didn't always feel like going, but I did. I planned on never having any regrets, and I don't.

"My dad developed throat cancer when my second child was born, and leukemia when my last child was born. He went through chemotherapy and radiation with the first cancer and was on different medications with the second. In all of that time, he never complained. Dad felt that you're dealt the hand that was given to you, you might not like it, but complaining wasn't going to change it, so deal with it. He didn't like to bother people about himself, didn't ever want to be the center of attention, and that is how he dealt with his cancers.

"He would drive himself to and from chemo treatments (an hour away in Philadelphia) when he had throat cancer. We always were aware of the illnesses but he never dwelt upon them. In fact, it wasn't until after my dad had a ruptured aneurysm, and didn't want to attempt the drive any more, that my mom even met his cancer doctor in Philadelphia. His cancer doctor joked with my mom that they began to think she was a figment of my dad's imagination as he had gone there for nine years before they ever met my mom.

"As I stated above, my dad had a ruptured aneurysm, and lived. That was a miracle in itself. After that he was never quite the same. At times, you saw his old 'zest' come out, but he was much more reserved. My girls often joke because they refer to the 'old grandpa', the one that spoke, and you listened, and the one after the aneurysm.

"After two years, and some other health issues, leukemia finally took my father's life. We visited his doctor on a Friday, and I had mentioned to him ahead of time that dad just wasn't quite 'with it'. Some things that previously appalled him didn't seem to matter anymore. That day the doctor took his blood, his platelets were at a low of 72 (average is 150-400). He had to be feeling *lousy.* This was on November 11th. The doctor said that he would be gone by Christmas, or possibly by Thanksgiving, which was in two weeks. He told me to call my brother in Chicago and have him come home the next weekend. However, my dad first had planned on going 'home' to upstate New York (we lived in South Jersey, 500 miles away). And so with a platelet count of 72, he traveled with my mom and older brother 500 miles home for the weekend. Everyone who saw him that weekend commented on his spirits, and that even though he was quiet, he talked and visited with everyone.

"Dad came home on Sunday and by Monday evening he didn't feel the best. I stopped over on Tuesday, and he mentioned staying in bed, but I got him up and onto his couch in his favorite room. (My dad believed that your health was more mind over matter. He prided himself on the fact that he worked for over 37 years at his company and never took a sick day). I had mentioned to him that his platelets were low and that his doctor had wanted 'help' to come in. He asked, "How low?" and I told him fewer than 100, as once again, I couldn't be totally honest, it just hurt too much. I explained to him that he was weak and it was a lot for my mom to get him around, so some help was going to come in for a few hours every day, just to help out. (I couldn't call it hospice because I knew what that meant and I was having a hard time dealing with it). Dad said the help would be okay.

"On Tuesday, hospice came in and he was fine that afternoon. In fact, a bed was ordered to be delivered on Wednesday and they didn't even leave medicine because he was so good.

"I brought him and my mom chicken for dinner and he was fine, but within two hours, when I stopped over again, he was groaning and having immense pain. Mom mentioned that this had started around 5:30, and it was now 6:00. However, forever my father, he didn't complain, just said it hurt. I was able to contact hospice and they were able to get me a prescription for Morphine. I went to the drug store while Mom stayed with Dad, and I then gave him Morphine three times. My mom and I sat with him during the evening. He didn't say much, his breathing was very labored.

"We learned later that the effort he was giving to breathe, where it sounded like he had something in his throat, was the *death rattle*. The woman from hospice had heard him breathing over the phone and mentioned that this could be the night, but who was to know? He had really only gotten sick around 5:30. Mom and I sat comforting him from 10 on, when he seemed most uncomfortable. He was gone at 12:40a.m.

"My dad died the way he would have wanted, in his own home, on his own couch, in his clothes, and it was very peaceful. He was not a demonstrative man but he was full of dignity and I think he willed his last hours. Once he realized his numbers and that hospice had come in, I think he just said I've had enough. He had been home, visited his brothers and sister, and was at peace.

"One of the first things I learned about him when he retired was that he loved the month of November, as the days are beautiful then in southern New Jersey. Well, Dad died early in the morning of what turned out to be a beautiful Fall day. He also was gone in mid-November, knowing my dad he figured, well if I go out now, it's a week before Thanksgiving, and over a month before Christmas, I won't ruin their holidays, and I won't 'hang on'. He would never have wanted to be a burden to us, and he wasn't.

"For a few weeks after his death, I wasn't content with how his last night had ended. When it first happened, I thought, WOW… that was the most peaceful, serene experience I have ever had. I had never been with anyone who had died, let alone a parent, but afterwards I thought, did I say enough? Did I do enough? Should I have said over and over, 'Dad, I love you,' but that wasn't my father. Yes, I told him that I loved him, but that night my mom and I were trying to calm him, telling him to relax and rest. Also, since no one actually knows when the end is, my mom and I didn't want to say or do anything to scare him. Could you imagine telling someone things thinking he had only hours to live, and then he thinking that, only to live more days, with the fright knowing he/she was dying? Dad didn't fight, but seemed to be at peace. My mom and I were with him at his last breaths, and it was very peaceful.

"I have come to accept that my dad knew I loved him, and the end was what he willed. He is at peace, with no more pain. I believe that he was probably in some pain those last months, but my dad, being the man he was, wouldn't speak or complain about it. I also feel honored that my mom and I were able to be with my dad. I have a sister who lives a few hours away from home, a brother who lives half way across the country, and another brother who is a widower and has a young son at home. I know they wished they could have been there, but as no one knows the end, and it happened so quickly, they weren't able to be there (probably my dad's wish to prevent everyone from coming in causing a big 'hoopla'). I hope, and pray, that I was there for all of us. My parents had been married for almost 56 years, and my mom and I were there to represent our 'gang' and show my dad how much we all loved him.

"My dad is buried in a cemetery two minutes from my house and I often stop to 'talk'. The pain comes and goes in waves, depending upon what is going on. But it is us here who miss him, but he is at peace.

"My girls all spoke at his funeral, a point that would have made my dad proud. In fact, as we all sat at the service, I instructed my girls (ages 11, 13, 15, and 17) to remember what their grandpa would have said, stand tall, speak loudly and clearly, and enunciate!! My oldest daughter summed it up best when she said, 'We all wish Grandpa was still here, but I believe that he is in heaven, smoking his pipe, reading his *Wall Street Journal*, and listening to Bing Crosby, with his dog Haley at his side (who had been hit and killed by a car two weeks prior to his death).'

"We should all be so lucky. And so, the man I admired most is gone, but I carry on, mostly do what he would want me to do, and hopefully, to live as he would want me to live, and to make him proud."

The Bond of Veterans

After stepping up the weather beaten ramp to my patient's front door, I scooted around what I thought was a typical recliner sitting on the front porch. When I entered the home, I saw Vietnam veterans with tattoos and burly beards attending to one of their own as he lay dying on this Memorial Day weekend. These heroes were there to ensure their buddy could join in the festivities on the lawn for what each recognized would be their last celebration together. I knew I was about to enter a land of laughter and cheer, despite the signs of illness that filled the home.

I needlessly voiced my concern over the discomfort of my frail patient sitting for hours in his wheelchair outside. Then I was asked to look closer to the recliner I had passed on my way in- the one with a scrap metal base, four heavy-duty wheels attached underneath, and a truck dolly strapped to the bulk of it. These *brothers* were the ultimate caregivers and creators of comfort for one of their own. I salute you all! Thank you for providing me the freedom that so many do not have.

Scenarios of Pain

I would guess that most of us have inadvertently listened to adult conversations and been involved in our family's activities that likely included discussions and/or activities relating to death and dying. Our comprehension of what dying is about, what behavior and responses are expected, the language used in relating to death, the rituals performed, and the values placed on the deceased slowly evolved. If we were raised not to fear death or dying but to understand it and maybe even embrace it then as adults we just may have obtained a *mature concept of death*. Realistically, our *mature concept of death* is liable to be fleeting if events in our final days or weeks of life cause us untoward concerns or anxiety, which brings us to what the majority of my end-of-life class attendees, my patients, and their care givers have told me was their greatest concern: uncontrolled pain. So I assume pain is probably what you would have also stated.

Whether we have pain that is acute or suddenly occurring, or if we have pain that is chronic or long-standing, we all want it at a level we can easily tolerate, but understandably we would prefer none at all. A fear some hospice patients or their caregivers may have is a drug addiction or dependence on pain medicines and thus a hesitation in taking medications may occur. Patients' medications are ordered by their physician without intent to hasten a death, cause an overdose or concern of addiction. Each medicine plays a significant role in providing a peaceful and comfortable quality of life at the end of life.

To best understand how pain can be anticipated and then controlled, I am using two scenarios that occurred with my hospice patients during the same weekend. This first scenario certainly and sadly could have been prevented.

Scenario #1: Lee had liver cancer and was cared for by his wife in their home. He had been a hospice patient for five days. His strength in providing his own physical care, administering the medications his physician ordered to control his symptoms, and voicing his needs had waned as he quickly approached death. So now he had to rely on his bride of fifty-five years to provide him his medications and daily care, as well as anticipate any unmet needs. She was not aware of Lee's medication routine before his decline and so, unfortunately, she did not understand the importance of Lee receiving his medications on a regular basis. She also had concerns that Lee may be over sedated, not realizing that his sleepiness was due more to his decline in health and approaching death than due to his medications.

While providing care for Lee, who was minimally responsive, I needed to gently reposition him to his side. During this brief moment of movement, Lee severely grimaced, moaned loudly and stiffened his body, indicating he was in great pain. Because his wife was present and observed Lee's very painful condition, a teaching-moment occurred and she quickly realized her error in judgment, so I thought.

With emotional support, end-of-life education, and stressing the importance of Lee receiving his medications regularly, his wife agreed to administer his pain medication while I was present, and the pain crisis was soon resolved during this visit. She acknowledged the need for pain control and voiced her understanding that the medications are normal doses, prescribed by their family doctor, and are not to hasten Lee's death but allow a better quality of life at the end of life. She assured me she would administer Lee's medications every four hours as ordered by his doctor, which is how often Lee took them on his own, and if she had any questions or concerns she would call hospice 24/7.

Lee was very comfortable by the end of my visit and I informed them both that I or another nurse would visit again the next day or sooner, if needed.

Very *unfortunately* for Lee, when I returned nearly twenty-six hours later, I discovered that his last dose of pain medication was when I visited the day prior! His wife had been awake with him all night and she stated she "was exhausted" and didn't know what to do, and did not call hospice. He very obviously was having another pain crisis and was extremely restless due to his uncontrolled pain, and perhaps imminent death.

Fortunately, their son who lived out of state had arrived just hours prior to my visit and stated he would gladly assist with his father's care and medication needs. So Lee's care needs and his medications were reviewed again with his wife and now his son, with both voicing understanding of all. However, there was some reluctance on the wife's part whether medications were needed to be given regularly and she was adamant that their son not be overly involved in his father's care.

My heart was literally breaking for Lee. I offered his wife around-the-clock nurses to remain in the home to provide support and pain management, plus I discussed the availability of the Hospice Care Center for Lee, which she said she had considered the week prior. Now she refused both. I offered a hospice chaplain and a social worker to provide more comfort and support to her husband, their son, and to her but she adamantly refused further assistance. Then she said, "He's not going to die and I don't want to talk about it!" Her denial of Lee's approaching death was all she could focus on.

My awareness of this elderly lady not being in the best of health physically or emotionally was also my concern. Her failure to provide intimate care for her husband was not because she didn't want to but simply because she wasn't physically able. Her anxiety over his possible death had escalated. She did not want her husband to die. He was her best friend and her life.

Yet, I was also aware that Lee may have his own concerns, not only about pain control, but he may also have some anxieties regarding his approaching death. He may have needed an opportunity for closure and to complete some unfinished business his wife may not be aware of.

Unfortunately, his wife would not allow any assistance from any member of the hospice team to discuss such anxieties and lack of closure on this day.

Lee died three days later. I do not know how his story ended because his regularly scheduled nurse attended to him upon his death. I fervently prayed until then that he would have a peaceful and pain-free passing.

Scenario #2: Thomas had ups and downs with his prostate cancer but one thing he had managed very well was the control of his pain. When he was admitted to hospice five days prior, he was already receiving pain medicine that he took every twelve hours, which is a long lasting or time-released medication. This pill controlled his pain very well. Tom also had a pain medicine he could take every four hours if his long acting medication wasn't working as well, which he noticed mainly when he performed more activities around the house.

Tom's wife recognized that he was sleepier when he had to take extra pain medicine but she was always able to easily awaken him if it was time to take a pill or an unexpected visitor dropped in. She was well aware of his medication schedule and needs and was very grateful for his pain control.

Tom's hospice nurse informed him and his wife that he may need to have his doctor increase his medication dose in the future as it was common to develop a tolerance to a routine dose and so it may not be quite as effective. Together they monitored closely for that need.

Tom died very peacefully three days after my visit, without pain or other symptoms hindering him, as his wife carefully monitored his need for medications and administered each when appropriate. She lovingly held him when he passed on to the heavenly life they both anticipated and openly discussed.

When You Were Away

A hospice goal is *no one dies alone*, but is that really what *everyone* wants? For those who choose to die alone, or in the absence of a particular person such as a spouse, we must honor their choice whether we agree with it or not. One Saturday morning, Mr. V. chose to die alone.

Mr. V. was a man fifty-four-years old who had been battling pancreatic cancer for many years. When I arrived at his bedside, he was in pain and having bouts of vomiting. His wife was crying softly while caring and comforting him.

Once Mr. V's symptoms were under control, I spoke privately with his wife about how sick her husband was and that I was uncertain of the hour or day he may die but thought it could be soon. Even though Mrs. V. cried harder, she knew the time was inevitable and her husband was ready to die. She voiced her exhaustion after lovingly caring for his needs around-the-clock for days and felt she needed to take a few moments to herself and collect her thoughts.

So Mrs. V. and I left shortly afterwards, going our separate ways, while their adult daughter remained in the home. Their daughter had spent many hours caring for her dad so Mrs. V. was comfortable leaving him briefly.

Within a very short period of time, I was called by hospice to return immediately to Mr. V. because within fifteen minutes of Mrs. V. and me leaving his bedside, Mr. V. died.

Mrs. V. was so distraught when I arrived several minutes after her. What I communicated to her was that it was probably his choice to die in her absence, perhaps believing his moment of death would be very hard on her.

In those moments, her only comfort was in knowing their daughter was in their home. Through tears, Mrs. V. shared many moments of joy she and her husband had experienced over many years together, and expressed their sorrow in awareness of his approaching death.

From Painful to Free of Pain

Patients in the United States are often under treated for pain according to a report by *The National Foundation for the Treatment of Pain*. As one who has worked for years in hospitals and with hospice, plus I have a large handful of friends who battle chronic pain, I would have to agree. Pain control is of utmost importance in caring for hospice patients. Hospice physicians have a tremendous knowledge in symptom management and work closely with hospice staff to ensure their patients have a quality of life with pain and other symptoms well managed.

Drowning in Morphine was a headline in an e-mail I got several years ago that made my blood boil. It heightened the importance of education as a critical component to ensure our patients and families feel comfortable in administering prescribed medication, including Morphine.

When Dad needed Morphine for pain and shortness of breath, I showed my mother the tiny partial dose I was giving him, and also the full dose he could have been given with the severest of symptoms, per his doctor's orders. I was required to document any medication I gave Dad, and the hospice nurse reviewed my documentation and compared it to the remaining amounts of each medication to confirm proper dosing. The documentation was always on the counter, visible to any family member who wished to see what Dad was given and when.

During one of my hospice visits, my patient's family members had just arrived from out of town and were so sure we were *killing* their loved one with Morphine, prescribed for her cancer pain, that they decided to withhold their mother's medicine. The family felt certain her medicine is what caused her physical decline and not the fact she was approaching death.

Within eight hours, she had a pain crisis that was off the chart. Of course, it took even more time to get her back to a tolerable level of pain, plus control her anxiety that was triggered by her pain and/or even the thought of severe pain re-occurring.

Another one of my patients was in severe respiratory distress. She became confused and forgot to take her Morphine which she needed for ease of breathing, not for pain control as she had none. Her caregiver did not realize her medicine had not been taken but soon discovered the need for and importance of it being given in a timely manner.

Even when my patient was receiving around-the-clock Morphine, she was awake and alert and able to carry on a normal conversation without any shortness of breath.

I visited another gentleman who was just hours from death. When I entered his home I knew it was wrapped in love by the butterflies that dangled from the top of the curtains near his bed, the Bible on the end table, the portrait of Jesus on the wall, and his very loving family attending to his needs.

Each voiced concerns that my patient acted painful due to his moaning and grimacing and he appeared anxious, restless, and "jittery". His wife reported that for years all he was used to taking was an occasional Tylenol, so his sudden change in his condition was of concern. She also reported he was no longer able to swallow pills or liquids.

Because of an increased risk of aspiration in patients approaching death, due to a decrease in ability to swallow pills, a doctor can order medicine to be administered in liquid, suppository, topical or other form. My patient's doctor had anticipated the potential need for liquid oral Morphine and so was available in the home, which eliminated the need to rush to the drug store.

After explaining the drug's purpose to my patient, who gave me a squeeze with his hand indicating he understood, then to his family, I was given permission to give some Morphine. I administered drops in his mouth, which did not cause him to choke.

Over the next thirty minutes, he settled to a much calmer state and was still able to provide some interaction with his family, even though he was only hours from death.

Toward the end of my visit, his daughter voiced a request, "You are obviously a Christian woman. Would you mind if we all have a word of prayer at Dad's bedside?" And so we did as calm settled over my patient and his very loving family. There is no better way to end my day.

Around the World

Pain is not always controlled here or on the far side of the globe. I was sadly reminded of that when I visited Indonesia in July 2006 with my brother, Gary.

During a conversation with one of the gentlemen we had met, I asked him if there was a hospice in the area. He had never heard the term hospice so I asked him where most people die. He said his mother had just recently died in their extended family home because they couldn't afford the hospital. He said that in order to stay in the hospital you must pay for your care and medicine on a daily basis or you will be discharged home. That is difficult to do when the average middle class salary in that area of Indonesia is $3/day. He told me his elderly mother was in severe pain until her last breath, with her family at her side.

Are we a blessed country or what?

Tell Me More About Hospice

To receive hospice care, an order must be obtained from one's doctor who anticipates a life expectancy of six months or less. If you feel you or your loved one is in need of hospice care, you can call a hospice organization yourself to get more information and they will make the appropriate doctor contacts, or you can ask your physician yourself. Your own doctor can be your primary contact and can continue to be the physician who cares for you during your hospice stay, unless the hospice physician is desired and agreed upon.

Hospice care is available in many areas across our nation and many places in the developed world so there is probably one in your area. Hospice organizations are typically listed in your phone book, or you can research the numerous resources available on the internet and some are referenced in the back of this book.

Most insurance companies provide hospice coverage. Also, Medicare and/or Medicaid may be available. A hospice team member, usually a social worker, can answer your questions regarding monetary concerns and, if not, can direct you to someone who can. No one should ever be turned away from hospice due to lack of finances as memorial funds are often available to assist those who have insufficient resources.

Make-A-Wish

The *Make-A-Wish Foundation of America* is a non-profit organization that grants wishes for children diagnosed with a life-threatening medical condition in the United States and its territories. The foundation believes that fulfilling a child's wish is a turning point for that child while battling their condition, giving them hope, strength, and joy.

Make-A-Wish International services children in nearly 50 countries on five continents with the same mission as their sister foundation.

To learn more about *Make-A-Wish,* and discover how to refer a child, visit http://wish.org/ or http://worldwish.org/en/.

Movies about Living and dying

There are some great movies out there that realistically place you at the bedside of the dying. Sally Fields starred in an excellent movie titled *Two Weeks* that portrays how her adult children adapted to her approaching death and the care they and hospice provided.

Another great movie about death and dying is *The Bucket List, f*eaturing Morgan Freeman and Jack Nicholson, a story of two dissimilar friends who live their lives to the fullest in their last days together. I like to see notations on Facebook and other social media sites when members state they have just crossed off an item on their bucket list. The adage is *live like you are dying,* as sung by Tim McGraw.

The Descendants, a movie starring George Clooney, is a very real depiction of a dying woman who had been in a tragic boating accident. Her family was confronted with decisions regarding her Advance Directives and end-of-life wishes that stipulate what our desires are regarding health care, estate distribution, and who we wish to advocate for us if we are no longer able.

Chapter 5 addresses Advance Directives and other concerns and, as difficult as it may be, it is best to make your own decisions before others are required or asked to make them for you.

4 Caregiving Guidelines

Recognizing the need and desire to be prepared for your loved one's approaching death is a major stepping stone in accepting the end of life. To ease this time of transition and best prepare you as you care for your loved one, I am providing you with some signs and symptoms that <u>may occur</u> and some guidance in how to manage them. It is my hope that you have hospice care to assist you with any needs you may have. Please contact your doctor for further guidance and assistance.

<u>Anxiety/restlessness</u>- The one you are caring for may pull on their linens, wander in their home, or toss and turn in bed, reach out into the air, and/or have poor quality of sleep or little sleep. They may verbalize their anxiety, which thankfully Dad was able to do and was eased with a low dose of Ativan.

How to help: Play soothing music and maintain a quiet atmosphere, sit quietly, hold their hand if desired which provides comfort in knowing he/she is not alone; make sure visitors do not speak inappropriately in one's presence as hearing is still present even if not acknowledged; provide a chaplain visit for spiritual needs if desired; provide a social worker if legal, personal or family issues may be a concern; massage, aromatherapy or other complementary therapies may ease symptoms; the doctor may order an anxiety medicine like Ativan or

Xanax to ease the restlessness especially if safety becomes a concern, if symptoms become more severe, or to provide needed rest; if he/she was an active smoker then a decrease in nicotine may cause restlessness and nicotine patches may be needed. The patient should also be assessed for pain, constipation, breathing difficulties, or urinary retention, which can all cause anxiety.

Breathing Changes- One's breathing may be irregular in rate and depth; apnea may occur which is the absence of breathing for 20 seconds or more; a gurgly sound may be heard in the back of the throat or breathing passageway; difficulty in breathing or shortness of breath may occur; loose dentures may obstruct ease of breathing.
    How to help: Reposition he/she to their side if able to tolerate it; elevate the head of their hospital bed as desired or use several pillows under their head and upper body; oxygen may be ordered if thought beneficial; a medicine may be ordered to dry up the secretions in the throat ie. Atropine, Levsin or Scopolamine; keep your home cool for ease of breathing and use a ceiling or portable fan; remove loose fitting dentures.

Confusion- The one you are caring for may be unaware of those who are in attendance, uncertain of the time, date, and place; words spoken may be mumbled or not clear in their meaning.
    How to help: Gently re-orient the one you are caring for; speak softly and honestly while listening to their concerns/needs.

Decrease in intake- As our body approaches death, the desire for food or liquids naturally decreases; skin may become very dry; nausea and/or vomiting may occur; retention of fluid, commonly referred to as edema, may occur in the arms, legs, abdomen, or lungs; increase risk for aspiration (ingestion of food or liquid into the lungs instead of the stomach) if a decrease in the ability to swallow occurs.

How to help: monitor for ease of swallowing and if unable do not administer anything orally until assessed by nurse or doctor; if able to swallow- provide small bites of foods like popsicles, jello, pudding, or sips of liquids, (cool temperature foods are generally tolerated better than warm); use moistened toothettes dipped in one's favorite drink or water to ease dryness of mouth; avoid using toothettes within the hour after administering medications that dissolve in the mouth; elevate legs on a foot stool or in recliner when sitting, place arms and hands on pillows to allow gravity to help reduce edema; apply lotion to dry skin on back, legs and arms, if desired.

Discoloration- Arms and legs may be pale, dusky, and/or have a bluish hue which may be referred to as mottling; one's skin may feel cool; nail beds and lips may have bluish hue

How to help: Provide a blanket, warm clothing and/or socks if desired.

Fatigue- The one you are caring for may have increased drowsiness and sleep more with or without medications; he/she may not be strong enough to stand on their own or transfer to a chair; may need to remain in bed; may be in a semi-coma or comatose state with very minimal to no response to voice or touch.

How to help: Let your presence be known with a soft voice and gentle touch; anticipate your loved one's needs that once were communicated to you; provide personal care and medications that your loved one is no longer able to provide for themselves.

Fever- A high temperature or fever may occur; perspiration may be prominent during fever.
How to help: Tylenol or Ibuprofen can be given orally or rectally if not allergic to; warm or tepid sponge baths are comforting and may lower the fever; linens and gown may need frequent changing; asses for infection.

Incontinence/loss of control over bowel or bladder- A decreased ability to release urine may occur causing discomfort and restlessness due to a full bladder; urine amount may decrease as the fluid intake decreases causing a darker, more concentrated urine color; bowel irregularity may occur as pain medicines often tend to be constipating and bowel activity decreases.
How to help: Contact your nurse or doctor as a catheter may need to be inserted into their bladder; laxatives, suppositories or enemas may be needed; have a commode and/or urinal available at the bedside if too weak to get to bathroom; use adult briefs if desired.

Pain- If pain control is a concern then medicines will need to be managed well; there may be more than one location and/or type of pain that needs to be addressed; pain may be exhibited through groaning, scowling, body rigidity or restlessness if unable to communicate verbally.
How to help: Administer pain medicine regularly as needed/ordered; if unable to swallow medicine your

doctor can convert the medications to liquid or an alternative form of administration (remember you are giving medications your doctor ordered to provide comfort, to promote quality of life at the end of life, and the medications are not intended to hasten one's death); call your nurse or doctor if any concerns, questions, or has poor pain control. Review dosages with family who are concerned with amounts given/needed.

Visions vs. hallucinations- Visions of deceased loved ones, heaven, Jesus, or angels may be spoken of; the one you are caring for may reach out as if trying to touch someone, talk about *going home* as they prepare for transition from this life to an afterlife; hallucinations with visions of bugs, dark places that are frightening, or other gloomy sensations may be related to a medication your loved one is taking and may be sensitive to.

How to help: Listen carefully to what one envisions and don't discount it as false; ask who/what one sees and share nonjudgmentally about it; if a medication side effect is a concern, please consult your nurse or doctor.

Glossary of Medical Terms

While all these terms may not be referred to in this book, they are common medical terms, simply defined, which may prove helpful to patients and families receiving medical care.

Acute- rapid onset with possibly severe symptoms
Apnea- a temporary pause/hesitation in breathing
ARNP- Advanced Registered Nurse Practitioner
Ascites- accumulation of fluid inside the abdomen

Aspiration- entry of secretions, fluids or food into trachea or lungs

ATC- around-the-clock, often refers to medication use

Bedpan- a container placed under a bedridden patient to collect urine or stool

Bereavement- state of mourning or sorrow after a loss

Blood pressure- measures pressure of blood against artery walls

BTP/break through pain- pain that occurs despite use of routine pain medication

Caregiver- a person who takes care of someone who is ill or needs assistance with care

Chaplain- a clergyman who serves religious/spiritual needs of a patient and/or family

Chronic- slow progression with long duration

CNA- Certified Nursing Assistant

Coma- a state of unconsciousness, with varying degrees of response

Commode- a portable toilet

Continuous Care- around-the-clock nursing care

Death Rattle- sound heard in the back of throat due to the accumulation of mucus that can't be coughed up or swallowed

DNR- Do Not Resuscitate

Drug Tolerance- a reduction in the effectiveness of a drug

Durable Medical Equipment- supplies that provide comfort and ease of care ex. hospital bed, commode, wheel chair, oxygen

Dyspnea- difficulty breathing

Edema- fluid accumulation in body tissues

Foley Catheter- a hollow tube placed in the bladder to drain urine out of the body

Guided Imagery- imagining positive images and
  desired outcomes, alone or with a practitioner's
  assistance
Healing Touch- energy based approach for healing by
  bringing one's energy back into balance
HCS/ Health Care Surrogate- a person assigned to make
  health care decisions on someone's behalf
Holistic- total patient care involving physical, social,
  emotional, spiritual, and economic needs
HHA- Home Health Aide
Hospice Care- care provided a terminally ill patient by
  an interdisciplinary team
Imminent Death- a death that is soon to occur, possibly
  within hours to two to three days
Incontinence- involuntary passage of bodily fluids such
  as urine and feces
Letting Go- the willingness to accept that death is
  inevitable and prepare for it, if possible
Life Review- recalling the past
Living Will- a document stating one's desire for or
  against the use of life sustaining medical care
LPN- Licensed Practical Nurse
Lymphoma- tumor of the lymph nodes
Massage- stroking/kneading/applying pressure to
  one's body
Metastasis- disease transfer from one body part to
  another
Morphine Sulfate- medication used to ease pain and/or
  breathing difficulties
Mottling- skin discolorations, often a bluish appearance,
  due to decreased circulation
Nasal Cannula- a hollow tube that delivers oxygen
  from a tank or machine to a patient with

the end of the tube resting in patient's nostrils
Nebulizer- converts liquid medicines into a fine mist spray to be inhaled/breathed in
PA- Physician's Assistant
Palliative Care- care given to bring comfort and ease symptoms, such as pain
Port-a-Cath- an implanted device that allows access for medications to be administered
Power of Attorney- a person assigned to make legal decisions on someone's behalf, if needed
Prn- whenever necessary or as needed
Respite Care- temporary care of a patient, allowing family or caregivers a needed rest
RN- Registered Nurse
Social Worker- assesses patient and family needs outside of nursing
Symptom Management- plan of care to alleviate a condition causing distress
Urinal- a container used to collect urine
Terminal Restlessness- anxiety/restlessness that may be exhibited in patients at the end of life
Toothette- a sponge-like swab for cleaning one's mouth
Vital signs- measure of blood pressure, pulse, respiration and/or temperature

5 End-of-Life Decisions

There are many decisions that we make throughout our lifetime, some impulsive and some well-thought out. The decisions we make as we approach our end of life may be the most important ones we could ever make. We must decide what care we want, who we want to provide our personal care, and to whom should we entrust the management of our affairs or estate. The following guidelines are to inform you of issues or directives of concern and *are not* considered a substitute for legal counsel and suggest you seek a trusted advisor.

Patient's Bill of Rights

If you have ever been in a hospital, health care facility, or a doctor's office than more than likely you noticed the *Patient's Bill of Rights* posted on the wall. Certain rights and responsibilities must be followed to ensure the best of care is provided to all patients. Here are five very brief summations from the twelve *Bill of Rights* that are written by *The American Hospital Association*:
1. The right to privacy
2. The right to Advance Directives
3. The right to make decisions about one's plan of care
4. The right to know of charges for services rendered
5. The right to considerate and respectful care.

The complete *Patient's Bill of Rights* can be viewed at *www://www.aha.org* which is the *American Hospital Association's* website.

Advance Directives

Through the *Patient Self-Determination Act of 1990*, the Federal Law requires that patients be provided with information on *Advance Directives* upon admission to a healthcare facility. In order to ensure one's wishes are acknowledged regarding health care and treatments, whether at the end of life or during an incident of incapacity, these documents or *Directives* need to be completed while one is deemed capable. Each document must be appropriately witnessed then copies given to those who need to know your wishes, including family members, physicians, healthcare facilities, and your lawyer. Any Directive can be revoked or amended at any time.

The following is a brief synopsis of *Advance Directives*:

Living Will- designates one's desire to have or not have life prolonging care during a terminal or irreversible condition or vegetative state. Desired care can be specific in regard to mechanical ventilation/respiration, use of intravenous fluids and/or a feeding tube, symptom management, and/or use of aggressive therapy.

Health Care Power of Attorney/HCPOA or Health Care Surrogate/HCS - designates a person or persons to make medical decisions and provide consent for health care if one is deemed unable to make those decisions for themselves.

Durable Power of Attorney/DPOA- designates a person or persons to make decisions for one who is deemed unable to make decisions for themselves in relation to property, finances, living trust, legal matters, health care, and other matters.

DNAR and *DNR-* are acronyms for *Do Not Attempt Resuscitation* and *Do Not Resuscitate.* A terminally ill patient who does not wish efforts taken to be revived if breathing or heart stops must sign this form, *along with their physician.* It is to be displayed in a prominent place in one's home, typically on the refrigerator, and in the patient's medical record. However, having this document posted in a prominent place in your home does not always mean it will be honored.

One of our patients, who lived alone, panicked and dialed 911. He was taken to the Emergency Room despite his DNR being appropriately displayed for all emergency personnel to see. He stopped breathing, was intubated, and the out-of-state family had to make the decision to remove life support, which they did because they knew and honored their loved one's wishes. This man died shortly after but the whole sequence of events could have brought a much more peaceful passing for our patient whose request was to die at home.

Organ or Anatomical Donation is the transferring of certain organs, tissues, or cells from a deceased donor to a recipient. This individual request can be noted on a Driver's License or on an Identification Card and be submitted to your state donor registry. If there is no designation of donor wishes but family members, HCS, or one's DPOA feel this may be something the deceased would have wanted to do then those with proper authority can consent for donation. There are further details at http://organdonor.gov/donor/index.htm.

If you would like more detailed information about *Advance Directives*, visit *Five Wishes* at http://www.agingwithdignity.org/, where you can also order *Advance Directive* forms that are available in twenty languages. Please note that at this time not all states accept these forms as legal documents. Even if your state does not yet recognize *Five Wishes*, it still provides a wealth of information to you.

To view sample documents specific to your State go to http://www.caringinfo.org/. Please *remember to use legal counsel to ensure proper legal documentation.*

Additional Documents or Directives

A *legal will* is a written document that ensures that after your death there is no misunderstanding as to whom you wish your estate or property to go to, who your chosen guardian should be for any underage children, and who the executor or personal representative of the will is to be. A will can be self-compiled or completed with the assistance of a lawyer. Using legal counsel to ensure proper completion and wording is highly recommended.

If the deceased did not have a written will then the State court determines how the property is distributed and, if required, who will obtain custody of the children. Some States allow only partial distribution of property to one's spouse and children before the court decides on estate distribution and may even place limits on access to bank funds very soon after one's death.

Unfortunately, the majority of Americans do not have a written will so one's end of life wishes may not be fulfilled and court decisions may be further delayed.

For more information on wills, go to http://www.aarp.org at the *American Association of Retired Persons* or phone 1-888-687-2277.

A perfect example regarding the importance of having a will occurred after the death of one of my hospice patients. This elderly lady needed someone to care for her during her last months of life so she asked her granddaughter to permanently move in with her. The grandmother *verbally* promised the granddaughter, who had several young children, that she would inherit her house after her death and so it was assumed that would occur. Very unfortunately, there was no will ever written to that effect. So upon an earlier than expected death of the grandmother, the granddaughter and her children came home after school and discovered the house locks had been changed, leaving them with no claim to any belongings inside.

Writing a will may seem like a premature thing to do in our younger years but it can be life impacting if not done, especially if an untimely death occurs.

Elder Exploitation and Abuse

The National Center on Elder Abuse website at www.ncea.aoa.gov reports that **elder exploitation** is the illegal taking, misuse, or concealment of funds, property, or assets of a vulnerable elder. Law enforcement officers and prosecutors are trained in how to use criminal and civil laws to bring elder abusers to justice.

Elder abuse can include physical, emotional, or sexual abuse, plus neglect in care, withholding medications, and abandonment. It is imperative that we monitor our elders for abuse.

A widowed and very mentally competent friend of mine, who I have known for over fourteen years, chose an out-of-state relative to be her DPOA and named on her bank accounts, and also on the deed to her house. Very sadly, this supposedly honest and trusted relative withdrew the elderly woman's life savings, leaving her less than ten-dollars in her accounts. Civil and criminal charges are pending against this dishonest and heartless relative.

Health Care Professionals are obligated to report any suspect of elder abuse, and certainly anyone else can. For more information, you can contact the national *Eldercare Locator* which is a public service of the *U.S. Administration on Aging.* The toll free number is 1-800-677-1116, Monday through Friday, 9am-8pm, except on Federal holidays. Your family physician can also be a contact.

If the situation is serious, threatening, or dangerous then 911 or the local police should be called for immediate help.

6 The Funerary Guide

Dying is like the sea, sometimes it rolls in gently, lapping the seashore without few ill effects, then changes into a roaring lion, battling anyone and anything in its way, instilling fear and foreboding. My desire is whether death comes slowly or at a moment's notice, crucial after care decisions have been made.

The time of our final departure from this life may be our biggest surprise ever. We may go before all our presents are opened, before the warranty on our car or refrigerator expires, before we have to renew our driver's license or passport, and probably before our grandchildren become parents or grandparents.

Perhaps death will come before the morning newspaper is dropped at the roadside, after the postman makes his afternoon delivery, or even as you sleep. Hopefully, someone will be with you, but remember it's possible you may be alone. My next patient, Jake, was not alone.

On the Edge of a King Bed

After kicking off my shoes, I crawled up on the king size bed where Jake lay on his left side. Countless times I have done the same maneuver but somehow this time felt a little different, more serene. His bedroom was filled with a sense of peace as if a burden had been lifted from within and yet saddled with an intense sorrow.

Glancing over Jake's right shoulder while kneeling behind him, I noticed precious family photos on the wicker stand an arm's length away and just steps from that sat a bedside commode. His very attentive and loving wife, Elisabeth, positioned herself at the edge of their bed she had shared for the last time. Tears were cascading down her cheeks from heartache and sorrow only a widow could understand as she waited for me to determine if he had really and truly died.

When married sixty-seven years ago in a little hamlet town in New England, Jake and Elisabeth would have never imagined their final days and hours together on earth would end like this. They never expected one would be providing such intimate care for the other and somehow find joy in doing it and compassion in sharing it. But with a team of hospice staff and volunteers assisting Jake and Elisabeth, he was able to die at home where he wanted, the way he wanted, and with whom he wanted. Plus, his funeral arrangements were in order.

To the skeptic, I say, "You are right! Death doesn't always look like this." None of us will die the same way Jake did, but most of us can die in peace and surrender as he did with loving arms wrapped around him.

Going to Heaven Soon

Mrs. T. was not afraid of dying. She stated up front that she knew she was dying and that it would be soon.

So together we enjoyed discussing heaven and how busy the angels must be preparing her new home. I didn't realize the impact our candid conversation would have on her daughter and two sons who were listening closely.

After chatting for approximately thirty minutes, I suggested to my pleasant, joy-filled patient that I may need to visit her the following weekend.

"Oh my!" she said, as she scowled at me. "I hope not. I expect to be in heaven!"

Upon leaving my patient, her daughter spoke privately to me outside the front door, stating how thankful she was that our conversation addressed her mother's dying. She said that her two brothers were having a very difficult time in accepting the fact and now they were much more aware of how close her death truly was and felt it was time to visit the funeral home.

Mrs. T. died two days later.

A Celebration of the Living

A Thanksgiving Memorial Service was my patient's last wish. He decided he wanted to be physically present at his celebration-of-life service so he could hear what others would say about him now, instead of never. He got his wish and it was a grand time for him as his family and friends came from every corner of the state to celebrate his living, before his dying.

Upon his death, his family told stories and laughed in celebration of this man's wonderful life as they surrounded him at his bedside. The tears flowed with joy and laughter, and in sorrow, while sharing in his life review.

What a tribute to a wonderful family-filled man.

I am not ready yet

The phone book was opened to the yellow pages as the headlines of *Funeral Directors* and *Funeral Planning* boldly lay before Jane's eyes. The yellow pages were slowly turning to blotches of gray as her tears toppled from her cheeks. Her trembling finger glided over the headlines as she kept repeating, "Why now? Why now? Why now?"

Instead of Jane being able to spend all of her last precious moments at her loved one's bedside, she was faced with perhaps hasty decisions in how to best pay tribute to her husband. Her decisions, that would reflect their beliefs, values, and familial customs, would be remembered and replayed in her mind for years to come.

If pre-planning for one's final care has not been done then numerous life impacting decisions must be made in just a matter of hours or a few days. Those decisions can include what type of service will be held and where will it be- in the funeral home, your church, or possibly your own home. What should be included in one's obituary, should you choose cremation or burial, which casket or urn do you desire, where should you bury your loved one or spread their ashes, and what will the expenses be?

Jane quickly realized the transition through these end-of-life hours would have been less distressing if only her and her husband had discussed these issues days, months, or even years prior to his death. With pre-planning, Jane and her husband would have been able to visit several funeral homes and decide together which one could best fulfill both their needs.

It is too late to offer some pre-planning guidance to Jane but it is not for you, so let us get started and get some answers to many questions my hospice families have asked about funeral care and services.

The Funeral Rule & General Price List

A benefit to Jane and anyone else faced with funeral decisions is a law that has been in effect since 1984 by *The United States Federal Trade Commission* called *The Funeral Rule*. Because significant sums of money for after death care may incur, part of this rule mandates that all funeral providers must offer the bereaved or other clients an accurate and written *General Price List* before final choices have been made. This list includes such things as charges for professional services of the funeral director and staff that are non-declinable, embalming and cremation costs, casket prices (you are allowed to buy a casket from an outside source, have a talented woodworker make one for you, or may be able to rent a casket for the service), an outer burial container if required by a cemetery, death certificates, use of funeral facilities, equipment and/or vehicles, graveside services, and forwarding or receiving the deceased from another funeral home. Purchases for single items can be made and/or a package may be available, which might include numerous ancillary items such as a photo collage, memorial folders, flowers, prayer cards, and/or memorial candle, etc.

Most funeral homes have chapels that are available for wakes, funerals, or memorial services. Typically, crematoriums do not have chapels. If desired, one's own church can be used for services instead of a funeral home and would typically have a lower expense involved. Many hospice facilities have their own chapel where hospice patients and families may choose to hold their service.

A celebration of one's life can include some very moving tributes and include some very unique items. One gentleman wanted his motorcycle at his memorial service so it was positioned in the front of the chapel where his riding partners recalled fond memories of their travels together.

Something that was common years ago, and is more common in other countries, is holding the wake and service in one's home.

Another concern is the cost to have one's remains transported a short or long distance from their town of residence or death to their chosen resting place. It is common for a funeral provider to have a transport cost considered as part of their basic service, usually within a twenty-five to fifty-mile radius. On the *General Price List* from a funeral provider, an accurate charge for transporting must be listed. If a longer distance is required, the local funeral provider can assist you in arranging transport, whether by plane or van, and inform you of the cost involved. Your local funeral home and the out-of-area funeral home remain in close communication so timely arrangements can be made with the proper paperwork and permits obtained.

If pre-planning has been done then, upon the death of your loved one, the first phone call should be to the funeral home where your preplanning was done. More expenses may incur with the use of a second funeral home so be sure to clarify that with your funeral provider.

A widow wished to have her loved one buried twelve hundred miles away where they had purchased two cemetery spaces years prior. She had a limited income and could not afford the extra cost of $950 to have him transported by plane.

So after her husband was embalmed, placed in a casket, then placed in her mini-van, their son drove north to their hometown funeral home with the proper and required paperwork and permits in hand.

Should I Pre-plan and Pre-pay?

There are individuals who are in favor of pre-paying for funeral services and those who prefer not to. Pre-planning is definitely advantageous, as Jane discovered, and it can be done with or without paying anything at the time of decision making.

The advantage of pre-paying offers less concern because you offset an increase in costs by locking in the price. However, that leads to my next question. What happens if your pre-paid funeral provider dissolves his or her business or changes ownership? When a licensed funeral home is to be sold, the State Regulatory Agency must approve the sale and requires by law that pre-paid monies must stay the same and must be honored. Remember that your questions or concerns are *free-to-ask* of your funeral provider by phone or in person.

Expenses for funeral services can vary significantly, even between funeral homes within just a few miles of each other. Just like any other important decision, it pays to compare facilities, staff, and costs. In my hometown, the *average* cost for cremation ranges from $800 to $1,000 and the *average* cost for a funeral service with embalming can range from $5,000 to $6,500. Certainly expenditures can vary depending on the services and items chosen, with even tens of thousands of dollars more being added to the cost.

Monies for After-Care

For those concerned about acquiring funds to pay for funeral services or medical expenses there are several options but you must carefully research each.

If you have a life insurance policy, you may be qualified for a *Viatical Settlement* or an *Accelerated Death Benefit/ADB* that allows terminal patients to obtain a portion of their policy funds prior to their death. One must use great caution in who they consult before deciding on a settlement because, unfortunately, honesty is not everyone's policy. Also, funeral homes will take an Insurance Policy Assignment.

For more information contact your funeral director, a trusted insurance agent, or research *The National Association of Insurance Commissioners* at http://www.naic.org/, which offers many articles relating to these topics. It is always wise to use legal counsel.

Another option in acquiring funds is through a *Reverse Mortgage*, which provides senior homeowners cash based on the equity of their home. Some elder friends of mine obtained a *Reverse Mortgage* through *The United States Department of Housing and Urban Development/HUD,* and are very pleased with it. Research http://www.hud.gov/buying/rvrsmort.cfm <u>or</u> call 1-202-708-1112 for more information.

Embalming

The practice of preserving bodies by embalming is thought to have begun with the Egyptians, prior to 4000BC. Through the use of numerous substances, such as herbs, salts, spices, aloes and wax, many have been preserved for hundreds of years in vaults. Eventually the practice of embalming spread to Europe then on to America where its use increased during the Civil War in an effort to preserve the fallen soldier who was a distance from his home.

Today, embalming pertains to the removal of body fluids and replacing it with a preservative solution. Embalming does not provide a permanent preservation but rather delays decomposition. It may be required by a funeral home for a public visitation.

A greater expense is involved with embalming over cremation because it entails much more. Approximately sixty percent of those embalmed are also cremated.

Cremation

Cremation, the reduction of one's body to ashes through the use of heat, has been traced back to about 3000BC. It was introduced to the western world by the Greeks around 1000BC when fallen soldiers were cremated and their ashes returned to their homeland. Cremation was also done for safety and health reasons when dangerous plagues killed thousands of people in the mid-1600s.

The first crematorium in the United States was opened in 1876. Not all funeral homes have their own crematoriums so they contract one in their area.

Nearly all religions approve of cremation, with the exceptions of Eastern Orthodox, Orthodox Jews, Islamic, and several Fundamentalist Christians.

Direct cremation is typically requested when no visitation or viewing is desired at the funeral or memorial service. A simpler casket made of cardboard is most often used for cremation. The ashes or cremains have the consistency of a coarse powder or coral, which are placed in a container called an *urn*.

When a service is held after the cremation, the urn is often positioned among cherished photos, keepsakes, and special memorabilia that represents the life of the deceased. Loved one's ashes may be spread *usually* where the family chooses, whether on land, at sea, or from the air, but if burial is chosen then purchasing a space or mausoleum will be an added expense.

State Laws mandate a waiting period prior to a cremation taking place. In the State of Florida, a forty-eight hour waiting period is required between the time of death and cremation. Your local funeral director will inform you of your area laws and answer any questions you may have about cremation. *The Internet Cremation Society* offers more information and includes pictures taken inside a crematorium at http://www.cremation.org/.

Caskets and Urns

When it comes to cost, the casket is usually the top of the price list for funerary consumers whether purchased at the funeral home or at a casket store. An approximate low-end price for a casket is $1,000, with much pricier caskets ranging well above $7,000. A plain pine casket can be purchased for approximately $600. Most caskets are made of steel, wood, or fiberglass, with or without a seal. You may be able to rent a casket for the service and then use a less expensive one for burial or cremation. It may be financially worthwhile to inquire at several funeral homes about the types of casket rentals. A funeral home charge for a casket rental averages $500-$1200.

If you have a carpenter friend or family member, you may choose to buy a casket kit, or purchase directions in how to construct one, and then have a casket fabricated with very loving hands. Instructions are easy to find on the Internet or ask for assistance in your local bookstore or library.

Urns can be purchased for approximately $30 but also have a wide variance in price. There are many different styles of keepsake urns and many beautiful pieces of jewelry that are designed to hold a tiny portion of ashes. A dove necklace of Barbara Graham's holds her mother's ashes, as shown below, and the urn crafted by nurse/artist Mary Freeman follows.

The funeral home must honor whatever casket or urn you choose when obtained from another source, whether purchased online, in-store, or custom made.

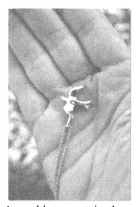

Barbara Graham's necklace contains her mother's ashes

Neptune Society

Over the past forty years, the *Neptune Society* has become the largest provider of cremation services in America and services over forty-five locations in the nation. One of the alternatives to a traditional cemetery burial is the placement of cremated remains in its Memorial Reef located off the coast of Florida. It is a man-made reef that is 16 acres in circumference and 40 feet below the surface of the ocean.

Spread the Ashes where?

A hospice nurse and co-worker, plus an amazing artist, named Mary Freeman shares a great story related to ashes. Bring on the joy, Mary!

One day my grandchildren, Little Charlie, Tommy, and Daisy, were playing inside my son Charlie's house. They were running their cars and trucks through a dirt road, making tracks along the way. Because my son didn't appreciate them bringing dirt inside, he yelled at them for doing just that. Then Little Charlie explained that he didn't bring in the dirt but got it from a bag in the closet. His dad soon realized it was his beloved Grandma's ashes. Charlie's wife, Dawn, took it very well because she said that Grandmother loved little kids and considered them to be a great blessing.

So they swept up the rest of the ashes and scattered them around outside where Grandma would want to be. Now don't you think Grandma had a hand in that?

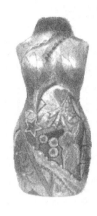

Urn Artist-
Mary Freeman

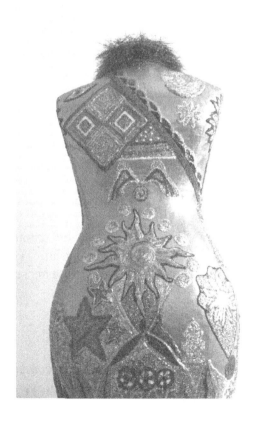

Facts on Cemetery Needs

A ground burial in a traditional cemetery has its own related fees that are separate from funeral provider costs, which may include a cemetery space and possibly an outer burial container. An outer burial container is a concrete container in which the casket is lowered into. Its purpose is to maintain level ground and support the use of heavy maintenance equipment without harming the caskets. There are no mandated laws that say an outer burial container must be used but cemeteries can require it. An average price of an outer burial container is $700-$1200.

A cemetery space can be purchased for a single burial or for multiple burials that will provide space for other family members. Depending on where the space is depends on the cost. I found numerous cemetery spaces for sale on the internet with the minimal single space price at $1500 then upward to $5,000.

It is important to ask cemetery owners about opening and closing fees, vault and headstone setting fees, ground keeping and perpetual upkeep fees. Some of these fees may be included in the space purchase but one should not assume so.

When a casket or urn is to be entombed in a mausoleum crypt, niche, or columbarium, (which are buildings typically above ground), various costs and fees also apply.

Green Burial

Green Burial sites allow for the deceased to return to nature through a natural decaying process at a much cheaper cost than a traditional burial. The deceased is placed in a biodegradable product that decomposes over time. There are numerous locations of *Green Cemeteries* and each must observe all state regulations and health requirements. Visit the *Green Burial Council* site at http://www.greenburialcouncil.org/.

Caring for our pets

Our pets provide us unconditional love and so it is very understandable that we grieve over their death. Many of us have taken our young children to the back of our lawns to bury our precious pets and hold a memorial service. These events provide us with *teachable moments* that begin the process of understanding that death comes to us all. It is important to provide closure whether through a simple backyard burial, to purchasing or making a specialty marker, or providing an urn for their ashes. Funeral providers and specialty pet shops offer an array of items for our pets, with many items also available on-line.

My brother Bruce says that if his dog Rocky isn't in heaven than he doesn't want to go there. Well, I most definitely believe Rocky is there and also our family dog, Spooky. Countless others, from priests to pastors to prophets, believe the same.

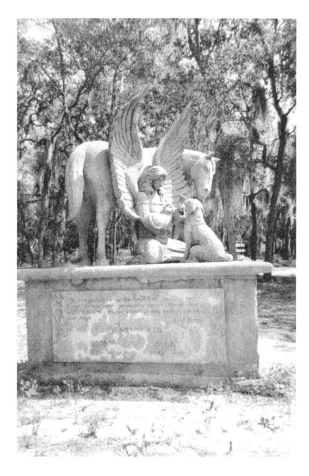

Pet cemetery statue in Central Florida

The Obituary and Funeral Forms

Upon meeting with your funeral director, he or she will assist you in compiling the information for your loved one's newspaper notice or obituary. Information you may want to provide may include your loved one's parents' names, immediate family members and survivors, schools attended, occupational background, suggested organization for memorial donations, personal accomplishments, and funeral or memorial service information. There may be an extra charge by the newspaper for obituaries and the inclusion of a picture.

For required forms and paperwork, your funeral director will ask you to provide your loved one's birth date, Social Security number, and Veteran's Discharge Papers.

Benefits for Veterans

All United States Veterans are entitled to a free cemetery space and one also for his/her spouse, an outer burial container, a memorial stone, and the payment of a Professional Service Fee. Active duty military honors are available to all Veterans. Your funeral home provider will have further veteran information and will be aware of any changes/additions. For more detailed information about veterans' funeral and memorial benefits visit http://www.cem.va.gov/ or phone 1-800-827-1000 to speak to someone in the *Department of Veterans Affairs.*

Another internet website you may find to be helpful is at http://www.military.com/benefits/burial-and-memorial.

The *Arlington National Cemetery* in Washington D.C.is well known for its availability to those who have served in the Armed Forces. There are over 100 National cemeteries throughout our country where veterans can be buried.

If you are searching for a burial location of a veteran and their family members in VA National Cemeteries, state veterans cemeteries, other military and Department of Interior cemeteries, or for veterans buried in private cemeteries with a government grave marker, go to http://gravelocator.cem.va.gov/index.html.

More information regarding burial benefits can be found at http://www.cem.va.gov/faq.asp.

TAPS/Tragedy Assistance Program for Survivors offers support for our Armed Forces surviving family members, who we should never forget nor the sacrifices they also made. *TAPS* cares for those left behind when a military death occurs, providing information about military grief and traumatic bereavement, plus support and compassionate assistance to those actively involved in survivor care. See page 160 for more on *TAPS*.

Acknowledging Our Veterans

My most poignant health care facility to visit was the Veterans Nursing Home. Inside those walls are men and women who allow me the right to live in a free country. I tried my best to always convey to my veterans, no matter where they resided, how very appreciative I was of their sacrifices and service. Their walls and dressers were usually covered with medals and pictures about which only they knew each story and what sacrifice it entailed.

I visited a soldier named Robert on a Sunday night when the love bugs (that really is a name of a bug in Florida) were thick and the number of tourists in town was even thicker, so it took me a little longer to get to Bob than hoped for.

During our time together, I expressed my gratitude to him for his valiant service to our country. Through his teary eyes he said how much he appreciated me acknowledging this, as so many won't and don't want to talk about it. Through his life review, he found a purpose in his service by expressing what he experienced.

Uncle Barney

When my Uncle Barney was killed during the Korean War, his mother, father, and two sisters suffered an immense amount of grief. It would take years before Grandpa would lift his fiddle again and Grandma to accompany him on the piano, as Barney played with them for most of his twenty-two years.

The memory of my Uncle Barnum Humiston was carried with me in every visit I made with my veteran patients. Certainly no one would have expected the news of his death in September 5th of 1952 to be delivered in such an unfathomable manner. My Aunt Donnamae tells the heartrending story about her only brother, my Uncle Barney:

Although it has been over seventy years ago, it seems like yesterday from the pain I have in my heart. It is very hard for me to talk about it as tears come to my eyes.

It was a sunny, warm day in September. We had not heard from Barney for about two weeks. He had been in the service for such a short time, around six months, so it was surprising that he was sent to Korea so soon. Troops were needed and although it was not called a war there was much fighting and many lives lost. Barney was an only son and could have chosen not to go to Korea but he wanted to go and get it over with.

My brother liked music and could play any instrument as it came to him very easy- guitar, banjo, violin, plus chords on the piano. He did all jobs on the farm and started driving tractor when he was very young. He liked cars and knew every make and model. He would go down to Bangor and visit Uncle Frank at the gas station and help him. Sometimes he would meet some friends there, of which he had many.

Before he left for Korea, Barney had just a few days at home in June. He told me that if he did not return to take good care of Mom and Dad. I think he had a feeling he would not be coming back.

While in the Army, Barney was a sharp shooter and drove a big tank. He was in the tank Battalion as a Private. Barney had one close friend in the Army but he went to Paris when Barney went to Korea.

During this time, Dad was working for a neighbor farmer and I was in grade school, which had already started. Shirley, my sister, was married to Carlton and was pregnant with their third child.

The morning we found out, I was sleeping in an upstairs bedroom. Mom woke me up to get ready for school. It was early. Dad had already left for work after milking our three or four cows.

Once downstairs, she opened one of the front doors, which we never used, because it was a very warm day and she wanted to let in some air.

I came down stairs and Mom said she had found a telegram inside the front door. As she read it, she said Barney had been wounded, and then she said, "Oh no! Barney has died…he was killed in action!"

We do not know how long the message had been there. The message could have been there for days. He died on September 5th. I turned thirteen on September 6.

Barney's body came by train and was escorted by one soldier. That was his job in the service to be with the family and with the deceased until the burial. They arrived in North Bangor, New York, and Barney was picked up by Spaulding's Funeral Home, which was in Bangor at that time.

The wake was at the funeral home and the service was at the Methodist Church in Bangor. School was let out for the funeral and there were so many at the church that there was not enough room so some were outside. There was a large crowd at the cemetery with military rites and a 21-gun salute with the bugle that played.

Barney was buried December 10th, on his birthday. He would have been twenty-two.

My Uncle Barney, who I never got to meet, would want you to remember that nearly 37,000 servicemen and women died in the Korean War, nearly 100,000 were wounded, and over 8,000 are listed as missing in action. It would be grand if a veteran that knew Barney would contact me, as noted on the author page, so I could share your words with Barney's only siblings, my Aunt Donnamae and my mother Shirley. A big thank you goes out to all of you who have served and suffered for our country so the rest of us can live in a land of the free.

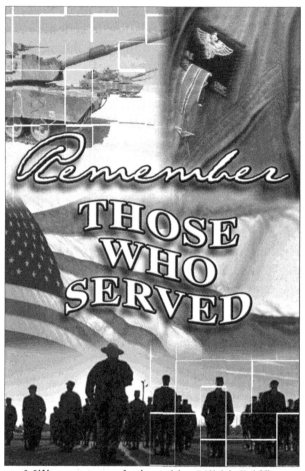

Military poster designed by Nikki Griffin

Funerary Artifacts

There are many precious items that come to mind when we think of those who cherished them and held them close: the American flag, Medals of Honor, jewelry, special collectibles, dolls, teddy bears, love letters, familiar coins, clothing, etc. Such items have strong memories attached to them and can be placed with the deceased temporarily or permanently, whether in the casket or during cremation. These precious items are known as *funerary artifacts*.

I recall tender moments when loved ones placed copies of precious photos inside a pocket, laid a favorite lap robe across their Mom's body, placed a golf tee inside a buddy's shirt pocket, tucked a keepsake doll under Grandma's arm, pinned a medal on a veteran's collar, put a favored locket around Auntie's neck, or laid a military dog tag by a father's side. The mother of my sister-in-law, Kathy Mackey Fairchild, requested her purse be placed inside her casket as she never was without it... and it was.

Dad and I loved an adventure! One of them involved making dandelion wine... comically Dad never drank alcohol, well, almost never. So, on the day of his funeral, held in the church he was one of the founders of, I tucked a dandelion in his casket, next to his elbow.

A Memory Box

Do you have treasured memorabilia from your loved one who has passed that may include old buttons, a broken locket, special coins, pieces of jewelry, a marble, or dice, a tiny doll head or stone? Years ago these treasures would be embedded in a putty-like substance on a vase or jar to hold precious tangible memories. Today you may find one of these beautiful jars displayed inside the walls of an antique store or in your family's attic.

One of my treasured friends has a wooden box that she keeps her husband's memorabilia in and when she sees something that reminds her of him, like a special card, she will buy it and place it inside her memory box.

I have a memory drawer. Tucked inside are a handful of treasured letters Dad had written and sent to me over the years. I also have several notes from my Uncle Dale. He was just like Dad, even their handwriting! Both loved an adventure and I am so lucky Mom and Aunt Eunice joined us in some! Both Uncle Dale and Uncle Jay sent me treasured letters about Dad's shenanigans during their years on their childhood farm. Is there a letter you could fill with wonderful memories and pass on?

If you have a special jar or box, maybe you would like to have it available at your loved one's service and request those attending to write down a special memory and tuck it inside for you to read later, during your own private time. It will be a precious way to begin your grieving process.

Headstones and Markers

The statue pictured on page 130 is located in a cemetery in Manitowoc, Wisconsin, not far from where my husband Paul's parents are buried. I do not know the one who sculpted her or how long she has posed there but her stone body shows many years of aging. There are no words to describe the emotion in her posture and face but I imagine all of us have at one time felt like she portrays.

In your town or in your travels be sure to glance into the cemeteries you pass as there are many gorgeous and unique headstones and monuments, also known as gravestones or tombstones, that pay tribute to those who lie below.

Personally, I consider the choice of a gravestone or urn, which will be viewed for perhaps centuries to come, to hold a greater significance for survivors than the casket lying beneath the ground that was viewed for a handful of hours.

There is a wide variance of cost for a gravestone, a marker, a monument, or memorial bench, as well as for pet markers. These items can range from a low cost of $150 to very elaborate gravestones of $100,000. Be sure to ask if there are any additional cemetery costs or fees above the purchase of your marker.

After discovering that a cemetery space and casket alone may cost $6,000, it is easy to see why an average price for a funeral can quickly escalate to $10,000. So why do some accumulate such expenses as they try to do their best in paying tribute to their loved one? I tend to believe we are emotionally weak and frail during our most intense hours of grief, and almost certainly in shock, so we may be less able to make the best of financial decisions.

When we are in our best of health is when we should pre-plan by making our funeral wishes known and, if able, pre-pay which locks in the price, or arrange for payments to be made over time. Either way, the burden of making hasty funeral decisions can be avoided.

Funeral Compliance

For those who desire more information about funeral planning and compliance, there is a wealth of information by *The Federal Trade Commission* at www.ftc.gov. Also at *http://www.funeralplan.com/* and *http://www.funerals.org* there are answers to questions you would never think to ask or think to be concerned about. Remember your local funeral home also offers compassionate care and guidance and can address many of your concerns. Education is empowering so learn all you can while you can. It just may save you some money and additional heartache at the end of life.

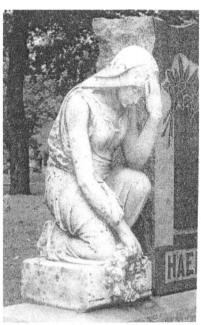

Statue in Manitowoc, WI cemetery

Organ Donation

One of the most solemn of moments in my nursing career occurred while I was working in the Operating Room during an organ transplant. You could hear a pin drop. The surgery was performed with a reverence I had never experienced before.

Discussing organ donation is a very difficult and emotional topic to address. There are sixteen deaths a day due to a lack of organ donations as reported by *The Agency for Health Care Administration.* Major organs such as heart, liver, lungs, pancreas, intestines and kidneys can be donated, as well as blood vessels, heart valves, tissue, skin, eye corneas, and bone. There are no absolute age limits in being an organ donor but you must be 18 years of age to decide for yourself.

It is likely that each of us already knows someone who was a donor and one who is a recipient. I met a woman who was given new corneas by grieving parents whose young child had died. Her gratitude and joy in being able to see her own children through the gift of another child was indescribable. She would like those parents to know how very grateful she is, as she has not met the mom and dad who so selflessly gave of their precious one.

The cost involved for the donor's organ transplantation is the responsibility of the recipient receiving the organ or tissue.

There are very strict guidelines that must be followed to allow for any transplant to occur. Certain diseases such as an actively spreading cancer, severe and current infections, or a diagnosis of HIV will rule out a potential donor.

A team of medical professionals must determine the absence of vital signs without life sustaining equipment, plus the absence of brain or brainstem activity. The coordination involved between transplant agencies, medical professionals, and numerous support staff along with the timeliness of it all is paramount to a successful transplant.

Leaving a Legacy Behind

Living donors have become more prevalent. When we talk about organ donation, it is common to hear discussions about a mother donating a kidney to her daughter, a lobe of a lung donated to a brother, or a portion of a pancreas donated to a diabetic child or adult. It is almost mind-boggling that our bodies have the power to heal others, as well as ourselves, yet we still must acknowledge the fact that we cannot live forever.

So, you have the potential to improve the life of a very ill person who has young children to raise, a daughter who needs a new femur so she can walk down the aisle, a teacher who wants to visualize her students again, or a teenager whose heart won't allow him or her to play basketball or soccer. Now is the time to have an honest discussion with your family and loved ones and tell them how you feel. Gather as much information as you can, starting at your Driver's License Office, the *Transplant Living* website, or at the *US Organ Donor* site at http://www.organdonor.gov/. What a huge act of kindness and a legacy for you to leave behind as an organ donor.

Autopsy

There is no way we can address all the things we have without briefly discussing autopsy, which is a very detailed exam of the deceased by a Medical Examiner who is a physician. Autopsies are done for various reasons: if the death is suspicious, to help solve a crime, for identifying genetic or infectious diseases, if the death is an accident, as part of a teaching hospital's curriculum to train physicians, or if the death occurred at home without an attending physician to substantiate the death. Once the autopsy is done, the funeral provider cares for the deceased as the family desires.

Individual Customs and Beliefs

One of the things I most appreciated while working in Operating Rooms across this country was that my patients were all dressed alike in their *gorgeous* hospital acquired gown, no makeup or jewelry adorned them, and a paper bonnet covered their hair. It allowed for all of my patients to be presented in a near identical way without any notion of financial or hierarchical status, and without potential for prejudice by anyone.

My hospice patients certainly have different needs than those I cared for in the Operating Room. Yet it is still without prejudice that I attended to the dying, their families, and their loved ones, respecting their beliefs, customs, and values specific to their culture or family upbringing.

Even though there are a wide variety of funeral and burial rituals around the world, each of them has a very similar goal and that is to show great respect and honor for the dying and deceased. It is impossible in this text to state the uniqueness of each culture because many have adapted portions of other cultures due to mobilizing from one area to another.

I would like to share some diversity of cultures of those who live within a short distance of each other in Central Florida and with whom I got to visit as a hospice nurse: at the bedside of an elderly gentleman who had just passed there was much emotion by his adult children with crying and pulling at one's clothes; while visiting in a nursing home, it was very peaceful and quiet as the extended family sat in prayer at the bedside of their dying father, each reading scripture from the Bible; two daughters in a small country home bathed and dressed their mother who had just passed, combed her hair then applied lipstick and rouge; in a condominium no one was allowed to touch or see the deceased after his death except for the nurse and funeral director; one evening three young children were lying in bed alongside their great-grandmother as she took her last breath; two grandchildren were taken to the neighbor's house during the last hour before death and the deceased was removed before the children returned

In every home I entered, it was imperative that I did not instill my beliefs upon anyone but honored and respected their choices and way of mourning. Universal compassion is paramount.

7 Coping with Grief

The way we react or respond physically, spiritually and emotionally to a death is termed *grief*. It is normal to exhibit certain signs and symptoms while in the process of grieving, yet each is uniquely our own and transpires at our own pace. *Mourning* describes how we deal or cope with our grief as we are confronted with our everyday responsibilities without our loved one present.

Those who are grieving and mourning after experiencing a recent death are often referred to as the *bereaved*. The ones I attended to commonly exhibited a blend of two behaviors in varying degrees:

The first behavioral response was a range of emotions where loved ones remained very close to the bedside of the deceased while crying tears of great sorrow, and even tears of gratitude that the disease would no longer inflict harm on their loved one.

Secondly, the survivor's behavior involved a more physical response with an active participation at the bedside with assisting in the final preparation of the deceased, tidying the room or home, and/or contacting those close to the family and friends.

As the hours and days of loneliness evolve, grief may be exhibited physically in various ways such as with shortness of breath, lack of sleep, sensing emptiness in the pit of one's stomach, shaking as if chilled, a change in appetite and/or tightness in the chest or throat. As the griever yearns for the deceased, he or she may be on a constant watch in attempt to see them or find them in a crowd, hoping somehow the death cannot possibly be true.

Psychologically, the survivor is forced to cope without the loved one present and may require fulfilling duties that are unfamiliar. The increased stress of adapting alone may even cause depression, despair, or a weakened immune system.

Guilt can be a significant burden especially if the death was sudden or if the caregiver believes it is caused by their lack of care or attention to details. One's behavior may change with isolation from social events generally involved in, wanting to talk unceasingly about the deceased, directing feelings of anger on others, and having waves of strong emotions.

Many grievers will look for comfort in their church or religious community. If one believes the deceased's spirit is present then that may help sustain them as they adapt and learn how to adjust without their loved one's physical presence.

Other grievers may blame God for their loved one's death. Followers may even move away from their religion, perhaps returning to it once the heaviest weight of grief has eased and a purpose or meaning in the death has been established.

An anonymous story circulated on the internet years ago that reminded me of what's important in life. I wish I knew the author, but it could possibly be any one of us:

A friend of mine opened his wife's underwear drawer and picked up a silk paper wrapped package. He unwrapped the box and stared at both the silk paper and the box. "She got this the first time we went to New York, eight or nine years ago. She has never put it on. She was saving if for a special occasion. Well, I guess this is it."

He got near the bed and placed the gift box next to the other clothes he was taking to the funeral home for his wife as she had just died. He said, "Never save something for a special occasion. Every day in your life is a special occasion."

I still think those words changed my life. Now I read more and clean less. I sit on the porch without worrying about anything. I spend more time with my family and less at work. I understand that life should be a source of experience to be lived up to, not survived through. I no longer keep anything for a special occasion. I use crystal glasses every day. I wear new clothes to go to the supermarket if I feel like it. I don't save my special perfume for special occasions. I use it whenever I want to. The words "someday…" and "one day…" are fading away from my dictionary. If it's worth seeing, listening to or doing, I want to see, listen or do it now. I don't know what my friend's wife would have done if she knew she wouldn't be there the next morning, this nobody can tell. I think she might have called her relatives and closest friends. She might call old friends to make peace over past quarrels. I'd like to think she would go out for Chinese food, her favorite. It's these small things that I would regret not doing, if I knew my time had come. I would regret it because I would no longer see my friends and family.

I would write letters that I wanted to write "One of these days." I would regret and feel sad because I didn't say to my brothers and sons, not enough times at least, how much I love them. Now, I try not to delay, postpone or keep anything that could bring laughter and joy into our lives. And, on each morning, I say to myself that this could be a special day. Each day, each hour, each minute, is special.

Pass the Scissors

The most touching visit for me is when I attend a husband and a wife at the bedside as one of them is dying. This is absolutely the tenderest of times, when two loves must confront letting go and saying goodbye. Even though most believe that heaven is on the other side of this life and they will be reunited in spirit, these last moments hold an immense amount of emotion, memories, and endearment. One visit in particular stands out.

I was in a home with a man whose wife had just died in his presence and their adult children, also. It was very difficult for them all to say goodbye once the funeral director was prepared to leave the home. The new widower had one final and very touching request.

The father turned to me and asked if he could save a lock of his wife's hair, something very tangible of hers, that he had caressed for more than fifty years. My thoughts immediately reflected back to the locks of my toddler sons' curls that I saved from their first haircuts.

So after I gently lifted his wife's head as he requested, he tearfully and reverently cut a lock of her hair from the nape of her neck. This act of love was a major step in his grief process.

Caring for Grandmother

Lying on the hospital bed with her face buried in her grandmother's pillow was Laura, the oldest of Mrs.

Em's six grandchildren. Her anticipatory grief was now realized as the reality and the shock surrounding her grandmother's death became evident.

As Grandma Em's body was removed from her home of eighty-seven years, sobs of sorrow spewed forth from Laura's throat. To her, the emotional pain of her grandmother's death was greater than any physical pain she had ever endured.

Within the walls of this old country farmhouse was where Laura had spent countless, treasured hours tagging behind her grandmother, making cookies, casseroles, and anything else they could conjure up for their family, neighbors, and those less fortunate. All that Grandma Em had taught Laura such as kindness, gentleness, meekness, reverence, devotion, and compassion, along with the power of amazing grace, would remain with Laura forever.

It was *filial piety*, a Chinese ideology, that her grandmother taught her for thirty-plus years. Grandmother Em had learned the same from her parents, which included the importance of honoring one's parents and caring for them until their deaths.

In those final hours, Laura promised her grandmother that her legacy would live on through her oldest grandchild and for generations to come.

Laura lay emotionally spent on her grandmother's bed with her head resting on the down of her pillow… and remained there upon my leaving.

A Messy Do

For nearly a dozen years I worked with Toni Porter at hospice, an awesome co-worker and friend who kept our hospice after-hours department together. Her story confirms that it may not only be the human spirit that can visit us after death:

My cousin's son died at the age of thirty due to heart disease. He was always playful with his mother, my cousin, and especially liked to mess her hair up.

One day while my cousin sat on her yard swing, watching her husband as he worked in the yard, a bird landed on the arm of the swing beside her. The bird hopped over to her by way of the back of the swing then jumped into her hair. There the bird ruffled her hair with his wings, stopped, flew off, and landed on the arm of the swing again.

Once again, the bird jumped over to her, landed in her hair, and ruffled it up. Then the bird flew off.

My cousin always felt that it was her son comforting her in a very familiar way.

A Swarm of Butterflies

There is not a sweeter, more spirit-filled woman and hospice nurse than Cheryl Maxwell. Her hospice families are very fortunate to have her at their bedside because of her great compassion and knowledge. I am honored to have worked with her for nearly all of my thirteen plus years with hospice, and call her my friend.

Just because we are hospice nurses and are familiar with the dying process does not mean our own personal grief is lessened. So when Cheryl's mother died she grieved her loss. Then several years later, she received a beautiful gift from her mother and God:

My mom, my best friend, passed over two years ago. I still think of her daily and miss her great, Godly wisdom. Every morning that I can, I walk the woods around my home. I enjoy watching the changing seasons and the wild life, plus it gives me time to think and pray.

On my daily walk I always pass by a large dead decaying tree that fell years ago during Hurricane Charley. One particular morning I was missing my mom terribly (to the point I felt like crying) and at that precise moment when I walked past the decaying tree, hundreds of Zebra butterflies swarmed out of the tree and encircled me for several minutes.

Needless to say, my knees were shaking, I felt so happy and loved as my mom loved butterflies and Texas wildflowers.

I look back now and realize this truly was a holy moment that God used to show me how near He and my mom are to me. I would like to think God and my mom were smiling down at my little girl's giddy reaction... such an awesome moment. Thank you, God. Thanks, Mom!

Hummingbirds from Dad

Shortly after Dad died, I went and sat on his porch, in his chair, reliving my last moments with him. It was just seconds from sitting down that a hummingbird flew into the window in front of me then flew away. I was shocked as I have never seen a hummingbird that far north, in very northern New York. Just as that thought crossed my mind another hummingbird flew into the window to the left of Dad's chair. Many patient's family members have told me of seeing owls, cardinals, or doves shortly after their loved ones died, a common occurrence. So, I am certain this was a sign that Dad was acknowledging our time together, a holy adventure I will never forget.

Precious Nails

Dena was a baby boomer who had been so attentively cared for by her sisters during her years of illness. So when I arrived at her bedside I anticipated a wonderful sisterhood surrounding this young woman's deathbed. Their sorrow was first displayed in the first hour after their sister's death.

Together, the sisters wanted to bathe Dena and then dress her in her favorite nightgown, a very pretty pastel pink. Then the sisters discussed the need to redo her nails, as Dena enjoyed having her nails look pretty. Each sister lovingly chose a hand or foot then gently removed the old polish, passing the nail polish remover silently between them. There was hardly a word spoken as they choreographed their moves. Then as quietly as that task was done, the small bottle of pink polish was passed between them the same way.

As each sister stood hunched over their youngest sibling, the tears of love slid down each of their cheeks with near-silent sobs of grief. I have never experienced such an intense sibling love for another through such a simple act that these sweet ladies exhibited. It is a scene that often replays in my mind.

Comfort and Hope

One of Donnette R. Alfelt's books, titled *Comfort and Hope,* holds some very reassuring and encouraging words for widows, widowers and any others who are grieving. Donnette, a widow herself, explains how the grief process may evolve:

It is the nature of grief to be unpredictable and undulating. If you expect a steady climbing recovery you will be disappointed and discouraged. It is normal for life to be abnormal for a time. I recall times of peace when I felt at last I had made it through. I also remember these states being followed by relapses seemingly from nowhere or triggered by some small incident. There are uses served by the grief process, even in the tears. Tears of grief have ingredients that differ from tears of joy or laughter. This indicates that they have a special useful purpose that should not be denied. The phrase "a good cry" is understood by anyone who has had one. As much as we sometimes resist or even fight them, there is a change in us physically and emotionally after we let go and let the tears come.

Helen Keller's Two Worlds

Helen Keller had many obstacles to overcome in her world of no sight and no sound. She explains in her book, *Light In My Darkness*, that it was her spiritual connection that helped sustain her through her sorrow. Helen believed there were two worlds. One world could be measured with a line and rule, and the other world with her heart and intuition.

Anticipatory Grief

Perhaps over a time frame of days, weeks, months or even years, the very ill and their caregivers have *anticipated* certain events to occur as decline and death approach. This *anticipatory grief* or expected reaction to a loss may begin when *little deaths* occur such as an increased dependence on others for personal care, needing to use a cane or walker, becoming wheelchair dependent or bed bound, or leaving employment.

Those who have time to plan for an anticipated death tend to have a much greater acceptance of it, recognizing the need of what must be done, the decisions to be made, and the time to make them. Stress may be diminished with a mutual awareness in knowing death is approaching.

Social Side of Grief

Many have explored the social seclusion related to widowhood. The bereaved is not only deprived of their mate but there may be a social stigma as one is viewed differently within their community. Thankfully there are many widows' groups offered through hospices, churches, and community organizations.

The Death of a Best Friend

My Grandpa Raymond died very suddenly in his northern New York home when his abdominal aortic aneurysm ruptured. Because I was very pregnant with my firstborn son, I was unable to travel 3,000 miles across the country to his funeral and grieved terribly over that. I couldn't understand why I grieved so as I was a nurse and *knew* about death…but it was years before I found closure.

Many years later, when my best friend Elaine died after several consecutive heart attacks at age fifty, grief again struck me with full force. I was devastated! Our sons were not only best buddies but she was my shopping partner, confidant, and co-worker. We sat side by side on the bench at every ballgame our sons played together. We would go shopping together every few months, often coming home with nothing. We solved all our problems together, and created some we didn't know we had.

Several days after her heart attack, I was informed that she was in a comatose state and not expected to recover. Some comfort came when my neighbor told me that Elaine had a vision of heaven after her first heart attack, which was quickly followed by her second. That was the first time I really thought of *near-death awareness*.

With my anticipatory grief tucked way inside, I got up enough courage and held back my tears long enough to *visit* my friend in the intensive care unit. The nurse was hesitant to let me in because I wasn't family. (Who ever made up that rule didn't have a best friend!)

Within a second of taking my dear friend's hand and quietly speaking her name, then mine, she became startled and the bells and whistles screamed out from the machines that she was connected to. Of course, the nurse rushed in and I was asked to immediately leave!

One very important thing my visit with Elaine in ICU taught me was no matter how "out of it" you think your loved one or patient is they just may be far more aware than what you may imagine.

My anticipatory grief was so severe I would not visit her again. I did not attend her weekday funeral as I had just started a new job and naively did not dare ask for a day off to pay tribute to my best friend. How stupid was my thinking? That is why I suggest you wisely choose the funerals you attend and the bedsides you visit. Thankfully, my husband Paul went to the funeral and offered our extreme sympathies.

Three years passed with me feeling sorry for my near friendless self. Finally, I decided that I needed and wanted to understand as much as I could about death, dying, and grieving. In my heart, I believe it is my way of honoring my friend by sharing my stories because I was not there for her when she needed me the most and I want to encourage others to learn from my mistakes.

I became an avid reader about end of life occurrences and found myself stocking my bookshelves with everything from near-death-experiences, to angels, miracles, and life after death. Soon thereafter I found the best nursing job I would ever have when I began working with hospice patients and families. I believe God had a very important hand in all of this, as my dear friend in spirit cheered me on.

A very significant part of my hospice life evolved as I began collecting and compiling stories told to me by my hospice patients and their loved ones, hospice staff and volunteers, neighbors, other health care providers, past acquaintances, and my own family members. Sharing one's story became a great way for all of them, and me, to find meaning and understanding of what we have experienced as one's death approached or already transpired. It has been also a great way for many to work through their grief by putting their story on paper…and having someone believe it.

Alas, I have finally reached a mature concept of death.

That does not mean I no longer grieve for my dear friend but rather I have accepted her death and have definitely grown as a result of it. I cannot physically see her but I can spiritually feel her as I joyfully recall all the belly laughs we had and realize they far outweigh the times of sorrow.

No Greater Love

The best of friends are undoubtedly those who are in a very loving and caring marriage, whether for five or fifty years, or seventy-five like Dad and Mom. We could learn volumes from them about loving, living, and dying. Studies have shown that the death of a spouse may even hasten the death of the other, perhaps this is grief's greatest blow. The term *chronic adversity* relates to this phenomenon of when the distress related to care giving of the very ill has a negative effect on the caregiver who may acquire or exacerbate diseases such as cancer, heart disease, diabetes mellitus, increased viral responses, and even periodontal disease.

Startling results from research indicates that the caregivers of the terminally ill may in fact die at a notably greater rate that those who were not caregivers. Two very devoted couples come to mind: In 2004, Superman hero Christopher Reeves died at age fifty. He credited his wife Dana's love and her care giving as to what sustained him far longer than anyone predicted. Eighteen months after her husband died, Dana died. She was only forty-four.

World famous singers/songwriters June Carter Cash and her husband Johnny Cash died four months apart in 2003. They were both in their early seventies.

My husband's friend and his wife died less than a week apart and shared in the same memorial service.

In my own experience as a hospice nurse, *chronic adversity* played out in one of my young married couples.

JP was twenty-seven-years-old when I cared for her. She was dying from cancer. She had a toddler son and a very loving and attentive husband. Just three months after her death, her husband died at twenty-nine-years of age of a rare type of cancer. He had no symptoms of the disease during his wife's illness or at her death.

Looking in the Mirror

My treasured friend, Doris, has been a widow for many years, but she has never forgotten the panic she felt when she realized she was alone. She also recalled looking in the mirror and seeing only pieces of herself and felt maybe she was going crazy. Even knowing that our separations are only temporary, there still are a wide range of emotions and symptoms to deal with.

The gamut of emotions can include fear, loss of appetite, emptiness, loneliness, confusion, despair, anger, depression, anxiety, misunderstanding, withdrawal, and denial. It is important to support our widows and help them to make new memories while they hold on to the old ones. We are instructed in James 1:27 to take care of our widows, as well as others in need: *Pure and genuine religion in the sight of God the Father means caring for orphans and widows in their distress and refusing to let the world corrupt you.*

A Child's Grief

Children go through a stage in their more dependent childhood when they don't like being alone so coping after a death may exaggerate their loneliness.

When a grieving child must temporarily leave their surviving parent it may cause a *separation anxiety*.

This reaction is similar to a child of divorce whose parents were both there supporting him or her in everyday activities and then suddenly one was absent. The memories may be too strong to deal with in those initial days or weeks of grieving so absence may seem the best and most secure option. In an end-of-life class I attended, I also discovered the same distancing reaction in adults who had experienced a close friend's death.

Additional signs of grieving, in a child or adult, may include nausea, lack of sleep, depression, general body aches, restlessness and/or shortness of breath. If a child or adult already has an illness then their symptoms may be more extreme, such as with allergies. When a child makes a significant change in their school grades, withdraws from friends, or wishes not to engage in functions they previously enjoyed, it may be a sign of grieving.

The Death of an Infant

No one is immune to the death of someone as precious as an infant, but nothing compares to the death of a pre-mature grandchild as Michele Milford shares:

I have often heard it said that God does not give us more than we can handle but, after losing my mother and father within thirteen months of each other, I thought that He was through sending me trials for a while.

Carolyn, my daughter, told us she was expecting her fifth child and was due in September, 2005. It was a difficult pregnancy, so we didn't allow ourselves to hope until she made it into the second trimester. It was as if she had flipped a switch and the pregnancy was progressing without incidence, so we began planning to decorate the nursery. I made a quilt with pale blues and yellows to welcome the baby that we had just learned would be a boy. His name was to be Matthew Alexander Woods.

Matthew was born at 12:41pm on May 27, 2005. He weighed 14 ounces and was 11 inches long. He never cried; he just lay in Carolyn's arms. He was breathing, but since she was only in her twenty-third week, the doctors said there was no hope for Matthew's survival. He was so small that the nurse wrapped him in a washcloth. He stayed in his mama's arms until he took his last breath at 2:49pm.

I never got to see him or hold him because I live so far away from Carolyn. I still have an empty feeling in my heart and look forward to the day when I will meet him in heaven.

The nurses brought in tiny handmade gowns for him and little crocheted blankets made by people in the Richmond area for babies like Matthew who are too tiny to fit into any store-bought clothes. This act of kindness touched my heart and when I returned home after the funeral I contacted the head of the Wee Care program in my area. My contribution is to embroider an angel carrying a baby on the corner of each blanket that is given to a family at their loss of a child. In this way, Matthew's little life continues to have meaning with what measure of comfort I can provide another family in their time of loss.

If any of you reading this gets to heaven before I do, please find my little Matthew and tell him that his nana loves him!

MISS

Attending an unexpected death of a newborn infant is probably the hardest thing I have experienced as a nurse. The air is filled with a sense of shock and an extreme sorrow. A surprising statistic shows that the majority of stillbirths are near full term infants with the expectation that, even with an earlier than expected delivery, each was expected to survive.

If you are a grieving parent, I recommend you find a computer and research the site *Mothers in Sympathy and Support (MISS)* which is for parents grieving over the death of their stillborn baby or infant. You can also call *MISS at 1-888-455-MISS (6577)*. Along with a bi-monthly newsletter, *MISS* also offers camps for siblings, educational seminars, annual conferences, as well as a multitude of links noted on their website that address a wide range of concerns that parents and caregivers may have.

To begin some of the first steps in the grieving process, *MISS* suggests both parents be involved in their infant's funeral and/or memorial service, the burial decisions, and allow extra time to provide special closure. Allow the family adequate time to hold their infant for as long as needed, which shows great compassion by the medical and funeral staff.

The importance of choosing a funeral home that is very sensitive to the special needs and requests of the parents is paramount. Grief counselors usually suggest that siblings be a very important part of the proceedings, perhaps allowing them to choose one of their own toys to be placed in the casket, provide the siblings time to speak at the service if able, and to carry the casket if desired.

Keepsakes are crucial in bonding the infant with his or her family. The baby's identification bracelet may be a very important keepsake to remove before burial. Making a videotape and/or taking pictures would provide memories of a time span that allowed few visual keepsakes. In lieu of flowers, the parents may suggest that their loved ones bring a stuffed animal to the service that can be donated to a favorite charity.

Parents in mourning are not only faced with immense heart break but often financial hardships, as medical costs can be huge and long-term. In regard to stillbirths, the issuance of a *Certificate of Birth Resulting in Stillbirth* can provide an income tax deduction that could assist with financial needs.

Other concerns specific to stillbirths and infant deaths are the need for medical research to decrease the incidence of infant deaths and stillbirths, provide funding for educating those responding during the death crisis such as paramedics, nurses, and police officers, as well as the need for bereavement support for the parents, siblings, dear friends and extended family. Any hospice organization can also provide a great resource for bereavement support even if the infant or child was not receiving hospice care.

Compassionate Friends is a nonprofit self-help organization that offers grief support for those who have experienced the death of a child. One thing that *The Compassionate Friends* sponsors in December of each year is the *Worldwide Candle Lighting* that honors the memory and the life of each child that has died. Visit http://www.compassionatefriends.org/home.aspx or you can phone 1-877-969-0010. Your local funeral home or hospice may also have a similar annual memorial service.

We are supposed to go first!

So often these are the words of the weak and frail elderly parents of middle-aged children as they deal with the imminent death of their adult sons and daughters. Their sorrow is as deep as if their child was young enough to sit and rock.

When I arrived at Katherine's home, tears streamed down her face as she sat on the hospital bed next to her adult child who lay dying. In my mind, I pictured Katherine as a young mother cuddled up in bed with her little one while she read her a bedtime story.

When I thought Katherine's strength to carry on was gone, she gently reached for her tattered Bible and began to read the 23rd Psalm. This amazing mother found strength in those final moments to share the comforting scriptures with her daughter: *The Lord is my shepherd, I shall lack nothing. He makes me lie down in green pastures, He leads me beside quiet waters, He restores my soul. He guides me in paths of righteousness for his name's sake. Even though I walk through the valley of the shadow of death, I will fear no evil, for you are with me; your rod and your staff, they comfort me.*

You prepare a table before me in the presence of my enemies. You anoint my head with oil; my cup overflows. Surely goodness and love will follow me all the days of my life, and I will dwell in the house of the Lord forever.

Grieving Celebrities

Does being a celebrity give you a special immunity to immense sorrow? Certainly not. A prime example is the faith-filled, Hollywood couple from the 40's and 50's known as the King of the Cowboys, Roy Rogers, and the Queen of the West, Dale Evans. Grief struck them their first blow when their two-year-old daughter Robin died from complications due to Down's Syndrome. Out of her grief, Dale wrote a book titled *Angel Unaware.*

Their second daughter, Debbie, who was twelve-years-old, died in a church bus accident on the way to deliver gifts to an orphanage in Mexico. She was once an orphan herself, as were many of Roy and Dale's children.

The couple's final blow came when their eighteen-year-old son, John David, who was nicknamed Sandy, died accidentally while stationed in the Army in Germany.

There are so many others whose names you will recognize who have experienced the death of their child: President George and Laura Bush, Paul Newman, Art Linkletter, Mary Tyler Moore, President John Kennedy, Abe Lincoln, Mark Twain, Marie Osmond, John Travolta, Bill Cosby, Jim Plunkett, and Eric Clapton.

How many parents do you think have had a military chaplain knock on their front door to bring them the news of the death of their son or daughter during service to their country? How many parents, grandparents, and siblings of children, who have died at the hands of perpetrators walk among us with hidden sorrow? I pray they find solace somehow, clinging to the joyful memories made together.

Disenfranchised Grief

Expressing our feelings about our grief may be even more difficult if it is not accepted or substantiated by our society, causing *disenfranchised grief.* If we don't talk about *it* then *it* didn't happen, right? Wrong!

The loss may not be openly acknowledged, ie. when a mother miscarries, has a stillborn child, or a family pet dies. Perhaps there may be a certain stigma that has already shunned the dying from our society, such as with one who has AIDS, has had an abortion, died by suicide, is mentally ill, is in a same-sex marriage, or an extra-marital affair. Any of these examples can cause *disenfranchised grief* that may delay the grieving process because there is a lack of support from a compassionate community or family.

Grief can be delayed even further if there is no funeral or memorial service to attend to and pay tribute to the one so loved.

Self-inflicted Death

Suicide...the word is emotionally painful just to type it. So let us make this word as comforting as possible when we talk about our loved one's suicide, as was suggested to a room full of bereaved during a conference I attended on grief. The grief counselor said, generally, we should say he/she died by suicide, not committed suicide. The suicide may have been a sudden impulse that could have never been predicted nor thwarted, an act of helplessness or hopelessness. Those are not a crime committed, but just a very sad occurrence. There is a difference between *died by suicide* and *committed suicide,* as in terrorist attacks. The latter is done by ruthless and coldblooded individuals, purposely killing the innocent.

The latest statistics reported in 2014 by *The American Association of Suicidology* lists suicide as the tenth leading cause of death overall in the United States of America, with most giving definitive warnings of their intent. It is the third leading cause of death for young people ages 15-24. The elderly have the highest rate of suicide at approximately 16%.

Centers for Disease Control and Prevention reports that more people die by suicide than by car accidents, and that for every suicide it is estimated there are six survivors, according to *The American Association of Sociology.*

For those seeking some guidance and a support system, there is a vast amount of information available online, plus your physician should be able to offer local resources. One of the main sources online is at http://www.suicidology.org/. If you are in a crisis situation you can call 1-800-273-TALK (8255) or call the *National Suicide Prevention Lifeline*-1-800-273-8255 or *SAVE-Suicide Awareness Voices of Education* at 1-800-273-8255. You can call about your own needs or on behalf of a loved one you have great concern for.

I can't imagine the sorrow of the survivors of those who died by suicide as they search to find meaning in a death of their loved one. Anger, guilt, rejection, shock, denial, and shame are just a few of the many emotions that disenfranchised grievers can experience as they mourn and struggle with disclosing very intimate information.

Whether the tragedy of an unforeseen death is related to severe depression or even an accidental death, we can all comfort those involved with open and nonjudgmental arms, and we can pray for them. We are not to judge them. We are not to point our fingers at them and whisper about them. We are not to throw a stone at them unless we want to throw it first at ourselves. May God hold you all close as you grieve.

Traumatic Deaths

Deaths that occur suddenly and senselessly can cause intense symptoms of grief including a strong longing and searching for the deceased, shock and denial, survivor's guilt, a rage against the perpetrator(s), and/or a severe anxiety that may be related to a loss of security or fear.

When we think of senseless tragedies and death there is no doubt that the murder of nearly three-thousand people in New York City on September 11, 2001 comes to mind. I wonder how many co-workers, friends, and strangers wrapped their arms around each other during their final minutes and hours, willing to lay down their life for one another.

My mind often reflects back on the tragic moments when many jumped to their deaths. I gained a better understanding of how those who died may have felt after I read a story about a man who fell a great distance while he was rock climbing. He fortunately survived his freefall so he could describe how he felt during the fall. He confirmed that he had no fear whatsoever, unlike those who were climbing above and below him who watched with horror, while the event unfolded. The climber described having a sense of being in safe arms as he fell, which gave him a great comfort.

Traumatic death goes on and on with the murders of the United States Ambassador and three of his staff members on September 11, 2012 in Benghazi, Libya, along with countless and senseless terrorists attacks before and after, including the Boston Marathon tragedy on April 15, 2013.

I recall the Ft. Hood shootings and deaths in 2009, and again in 2014.

Just days before Christmas in 2012, twenty young children and six adults from the Sandy Hook Elementary School in Connecticut were murdered. It is impossible to fathom the sorrow that engulfed their families and community.

Memories continue as I recall the Indian Ocean earthquake on December 26, 2004 that killed some 230,000 people across a handful of countries, and the earthquake and tsunami striking Japan on March 11, 2011 that killed nearly 19,000 people.

I remember the aerial disaster of the TWA flight on July 17, 1996 that exploded and crashed shortly after take-off from John F. Kennedy Airport with 230 passengers and crew on-board. The most recent aerial disaster is the disappearance of the Malaysian airliner on March 8, 2014 that carried 239 passengers and crew on-board.

Tragedy continued with the March 22nd mud slide in the State of Washington, killing at least thirty with loved ones still unaccounted for.

Off the coast of South Korea, a ferry sank on April 16, 2014 carrying nearly 300 young people to their deaths. Just weeks later, hundreds of miners died in an explosion in a Turkey coal mine.

Since moving to Florida in 1982, I have watched in awe as rockets and space shuttles soared over the Atlantic

Ocean. So the explosions of the Columbia on February 1, 2003 and the Challenger on January 28, 1986 are embedded in my memory. The exuberance and expressions of joy that loved ones displayed live on TV quickly turned to disbelief and deep sorrow.

How do all these survivors cope and find meaning, if there is any, with the shock and grief surrounding traumatic deaths? The overwhelmed survivor, who includes the first responders, may have delayed grief, requiring a longer period of time to process the incomprehensibility of the tragedies and deaths that have occurred.

With multiple deaths, bereavement overload may be experienced as the survivor attempts to grieve for so many at the same time. The elderly who have experienced the deaths of many family members and friends are also faced with bereavement overload, while anticipating their own death.

The U.S. Department of Health and Human Services offers ways of coping and dealing with traumatic events. You can phone 1-877-696-6775 or visit http://www.hhs.gov/disasters/emergency/mentalhealth/index.html.

Your local hospice is available to assist all those who are grieving, not only their patients and families. Your local church should have support contacts, as well.

World of Wars

The thousands upon thousands of deaths of the world's servicemen and women who have fought, suffered, and died, and many who disappeared in the wars and so-called conflicts, have affected thousands upon thousands more. The survivors and their loved ones must assuredly be changed forever.

There are a number of great resources available for our military families. The *Wounded Warrior Project* helps injured service members and their families through their recovery. The project helps move them from "surviving" to "thriving" over their visible and invisible injuries. Their website is https://support. woundedwarriorproject.org/.

On page 122, I referred to TAPS- *Tragedy Assistance Program for Survivors,* the non-profit Veteran Service Organization that offers a great support system for the *survivors* of those who have served in the Armed Forces. Because these families may have to relocate immediately from their home base of service, their support system of friends and military neighbors are left behind. TAPS can become a valuable asset through the use of their caseworkers, videos, magazines, grief camps and retreats, support groups, plus many other ways it provides hope and healing as families mourn. Their website is http://www.taps.org/ or you can call them at 1-800-959-TAPS(8277) for more information and assistance.

In Memory of John Ruffin

Tragedy may be closer than we realize as hospice nurse Linda Neider discovered on her birthday:

It was September 9, 2000, my fiftieth birthday. I received a telephone call at 5a.m. from my daughter Tara who said, "We are on our way, Mom."

My daughter, son-in-law, and granddaughter were coming to Florida from North Carolina to celebrate my birthday and to take our granddaughter to some of the places we had taken Tara when she was a little girl

At 5:20a.m., we received another call, "Mom, John is dead!"

"What do you mean?" I asked in disbelief.

"He's dead, Mom. We were hit! I have got to go to the hospital now!" And she hung up.

My husband Dan was already up and sitting at the kitchen table, as he intuitively knew when that second call came it was not good news. We made a few phone calls, readied ourselves for the trip ahead, and left shortly after for North Carolina.

It seemed like it was the longest trip we ever made. We could not talk or listen to the radio. We had to hold it together to get there safely. We were in shock and saddened by the news of John's death, and so grateful at the same time that the girls were not harmed. What comfort could we possibly provide to David and Faye, John's parents, whose only child had been taken by death? It was a tough drive.

We arrived in North Carolina approximately nine hours later. With my daughter in my arms, she exclaimed, "I have had my butt kicked, Mom!" (Tara had the idea that she was ten feet tall and bulletproof).

Many of John's relatives had already arrived and we were told about the circumstances of the accident. The car was hit from behind while sitting at a traffic light just after John and Tara had gotten gas for the trip.

Tara told us how she tried to get John out of the car but could not get the window open. She had felt John and he was soft and warm and she thought he was alive and just unconscious.

The rescue people had arrived on the scene and she yelled to them to help her get him out because she knew CPR. By the time she got to John, she knew it was too late.

She said, "I just took him in my arms and held him and told him how much I loved him!"

The funeral was held on September 11. It was a beautiful service and they played Vince Gill's song *Go Rest High On That Mountain.* John's dad took Jesus into his life that day, as did many others.

On the road to the cemetery, I noticed all the police officers that were posted to escort the procession had their hats placed over their hearts. I was deeply moved and comforted by this, as I am sure everyone else was.

When we arrived back at John's parents' home, Faye told us that one of the rescue persons had come by to tell her this: "When we arrived on the scene of the accident, we saw a light around the woman and the child, like a halo type light!"

This declaration gave much comfort to all. In my heart I believe it was John's light, as I knew how much and how deeply he loved Tara and Auslynn. I believe he could not have left this world without knowing they were all right.

With heavy hearts, Dan and I knew we had to return to Florida. We bid our farewells with the promise that I would return as often and as soon as I could to just be there through the next year.

On the way home, we were still unable to talk much or play the radio. When we hit the Florida Sate line, we decided to put the radio on and much to our surprise the song that was playing was Vince Gill's *Go Rest High On That Mountain.*

As a hospice nurse, I have seen the gifts built into the dying process that comfort the ones left behind when the patient dies. I have often wondered if these gifts were provided with sudden death. I now believe they are.

About six weeks after John died, my daughter told me of an experience she had one night. She was very depressed and was begging to see John one more time. She wanted to feel him one more time, hold him one more time. She said she woke up somewhere around 3a.m. and she could see John standing in the doorway of her bedroom. She went to him and he held her in his arms. She said, "Mom, I could feel his warmth. I could even smell him, and I knew everything would be okay."

Linda adds, "This experience gave her more comfort then I can describe. It gave her strength to go on and it gave her peace. Be aware of how precious life really is and that every life is a gift and could be gone tomorrow. Whether it is a life ending disease or sudden tragic death, death teaches us how to live if we but listen. Death is the great equalizer, it has no boundaries, and it is the one sure thing we all have in common."

The Empty Chair

When my best friend died, my love and friendship for her did not die but rather she became more precious on a different level. In order for me to continue on, I had to relocate her from my physical life into my spiritual life.

The empty chair at your family's table will forever be empty and it will be a constant reminder of your loss. Grief counselors suggest there is healing power in talking to that empty chair, or it may be to a headstone or a picture, as if your loved one is right there with you. It can be very cleansing whether you cry and/or get angry, or whatever your emotion, as that may be part of your grieving which is uniquely yours.

A Farewell Letter

There is power in the written word and so letter writing may comfort those that mourn. Having the opportunity to say words that were too hard to say before and no time to say them, to ask for forgiveness, or to say goodbye can give you some closure that is intimately yours. You can tuck it inside your loved one's pocket in the casket or toss into the embers of a fire.

From a Cocoon to a Butterfly

As part of my nurse's training in the early seventies, I was required to read the book *On Death and Dying* published in 1969 by internationally renowned author Dr. Elisabeth Kubler-Ross. She said that our patients will tell us everything we need to know about when they are going to die so we must listen carefully.

I discovered her tremendous compassion for those approaching death and studied her well-known five stages of dying, which include denial, anger, bargaining, depression, and acceptance, which have been discussed and debated for years and will continue to be for many more. After her stroke left her incapacitated, Elisabeth recognized that there was indeed a sixth stage, when she was angry at God.

When Elisabeth was volunteering in a post-World War II concentration camp in 1945, she discovered that children had carved butterflies in the walls just prior to entering the gas chambers; thus the butterfly became her symbol that demonstrated that no matter how severe one's life circumstances are, we can have a beautiful and spiritual transformation from this life to the next.

Her legacy to us is her transforming of end-of-life care around the world and being an outspoken advocate on the behalf of the dying. She died on August 24, 2004 at the age of seventy-eight.

St. Christopher's Hospice

In 1967, Dame Cicely Saunders founded the world-renowned international hospice training facility called *St. Christopher's Hospice* near London, England, which I was so blessed to have been able to visit in September 2004.

Her holistic approach in caring for the dying addressed not only her patients' physical needs but also their spiritual, psychosocial and familial needs. She undoubtedly understood the needs of the dying, the depth of sorrow that surrounds them, and the burdens carried by the caregivers. She also understood and recognized how important it was to instill joy at the bedside of the dying in her facility, on the campus grounds, and in patients' homes.

Cicely felt that humans cannot come to maturity until they have faced distress and that the ones we turn to in our time of sorrow, the ones who can understand us the best, is those who have already endured it.

Cicely died on July 14, 2005 just before her eighty-seventh birthday.

The greatest of thanatologists, those who are specialists in death and dying, are by far my patients. Each has made me more compassionate and understanding of what truly is needed as death approaches. They have taught me not to fear death but empowered me to seek the joy that is plentiful even at the bedside of the dying.

Anger and Endurance

One's approaching death may require a tremendous endurance on the patient and caregiver's part, as it can occur within two minutes, two hours, two days, two months, or two years from when it was initially predicted to occur. It is impossible to fathom the burden carried by loved ones as they walk down hallways with their heads bowed low, shoulders slumped, feet barely lifting from one step to the next, while they make their way to the bedsides of loved ones who are dying, and finally to the empty bed.

Because caring for the dying involves not just providing for their physical needs, it is paramount that one anticipate their loved ones unmet emotional and spiritual needs, as well. Their anger and frustration may become overwhelming and may be echoed onto those around them. This is certainly understandable. That is why the teamwork of hospice staff, including social workers and chaplains, is such an important aspect of end-of-life care.

I encourage you to study and learn all you can from those who have traveled through life with the dying and with those who are grieving. There are countless resources available on the web or at your library, numerous death education courses available at many colleges and universities, and many associations and organizations that address the needs of the dying and those bereaved…many you will find referenced in the back of the book.

Seeking You in Death

As I sit and watch the night fall
My arms ache to hold you
My spirit touches my sorrow

I was told breathing is living
Yet mine is so labored
And I am weakened

An inner storm is surging
The power of thunder is present
Yet the air is silent

I turn toward a familiar voice,
A familiar walk, a familiar laugh
But each is not yours

Sleep well in heaven, my love
Where there are no more tears
And no more sorrow

You are my star, shining bright
You are my champion, so strong
You are with Him now

But will always be mine

by Judy Voss

My brother, Gary Fairchild, wrote and read the following to a packed church, with standing room only, at our Dad's funeral. I am so thankful to have his permission to share what he so eloquently wrote:

My Dad

Dad was a farmer. He loved being a farmer. He loved making maple syrup in the early spring, tapping trees and boiling sap in his home-made evaporator and the sight of steam billowing from the sugar house. He loved spring's work and the smell of freshly turned sod. He loved the sight of the shoots of corn just emerging from the earth. He loved to walk through the rows of corn when it was knee high, his hands gently touching the leaves. He loved haying, cutting hay and baling hay. (Picking up the bales, stacking them on the wagon and drawing them to the barn-not so much.) He loved to chop corn and the smell of ensilage being blown into the silo. He loved the feel and smell of the barn, full of fodder in the fall when the cows went into the barn for the winter. He loved to milk cows, the sound of the pulsating milking machines, the roar of the compressor in the cold winter night air. He loved to farm.

He loved Mom. He and Mom were a team. I remember when I was small, Mom starting the afternoon chores when Dad was working at the GLF before he became a full-time farmer. In my college years, there were dorm room debates about woman's liberation and their inferior position to men in our culture. Maybe it was my males insensitively, but that was not my perception of my Dad and Mom. They were equal members of the same team. They played different positions, but were equal, in my young eyes. And, Dad loved Mom profoundly.

He loved his children, each one of us for who we were, and who we became. He encouraged me to pursue my dreams, as I am sure he did with my siblings. He gave us the confidence to step out into the world to make it on our own. What an invaluable gift.

Dad loved this church he helped build. He loved the people of this church. He and Mom brought us here every Sunday. That too he did for his family's spiritual development.

He loved God. I remember sneaking down the stairs peeking through the door or trying to listen through the floor register to hear him pray for each of us before they went to bed when we lived in the house on the home place.

He loved his community: the school, his neighbors, his siblings. He loved going on rides on Sunday afternoons "up south", pointing out to us his roots.

He loved visiting cemeteries. He told me once looking at the grave stones these are my people.

From about age 8, I began helping Dad in the barn, carrying pales full of milk to the milk house. During those days, I would talk to him. I think I must have been an incessant talker. He was patient and kind to listen. As I grew, we conversed about every subject you can imagine: great long discussions about life and God and everything else. That lasted every day for about 10 years. That is a lot of time for a Dad to spend with his son. It was the greatest gift he ever gave to me. Those years of hours being with him affect me to this day.

When I left home the physical distance between us grew, until half a world separated us. From then on, I missed much of his life and he missed much of mine. But the example of his life never left me and the life lessons I learned from him enabled me to navigate the world and live anywhere. By the way, when I told my Indonesian friends he was a farmer, they assumed he was rich. I did not tell them differently.

Thank you, Dad, for loving Mom, for loving your family, for loving your grandchildren and great-grandchildren, for loving my family, for loving God, for loving your church, for loving your community and for loving being a farmer.

Finally, thank you to all the doctors and nurses that cared for Dad in Malone, Burlington, and Potsdam hospitals. Thanks to the neighbors who stopped by often just to say "hi" and to chat a while and thank you to the caregivers and house cleaners and so many others that I don't even know and have never met that made Dad's last days as easy and pain free as possible. Thank you, Donnamae, for being a great sister-in-law. Thanks sister Kathy for your many trips from Syracuse to spend weekends at home with Dad and Mom. Thank you, Judy, for your special care. And especially thanks to Brian and Kathy and Beth and Earl for carrying the lion's share of Dad and Mom's care for the past several years. For all of you, I am deeply grateful.

Reflections on Joy and Sorrow
My Time With My Dad

Just because I may be more familiar with death and dying than someone else doesn't make my acceptance of death any easier or my sorrow any less. But while caring for Dad, I tried not to dwell on the sorrow but savor the immense joy of being with him, caring for him, making sure his passing was peaceful and pain free.

Dad knew me longer than anyone else in my life. I loved the farm and always preferred to be outside or in the barn with him. We were great pals and adventure seekers; we traveled to so many places, Dad, Mom, and me. He confided his health concerns with me as I questioned him closely and he often had questions for Paul, my pharmacist husband, about what meds he needed and should take. Dad and I spent many days and nights together in hospitals through many of his severest illnesses. I expect the doctors and nurses thought I was a gloating daughter but who else would ensure his comfort as well as I? Dad loved his family, his friends, his farm, his church and Jesus. I admired his will to live to 100, making it just shy of 97, and especially his unconditional love for everyone, something I struggle to have.

Dad's last adventure he requested from me was just hours before he died. He said, "I want to go fishing." It saddened me greatly then, and for days, that I couldn't fulfill his last wish for adventure. But then I found my solace in one thing- Dad's joy in fishing with Jesus and his brothers on the heavenly Sea of Galilee.

Many did not know Dad was blind in one eye for many years, and had very, very poor vision in the other, especially in his final days. He often recognized people by their voice, not by sight. He was so afraid of going blind. I know Dad was so afraid of dying, too, that caused his greatest anxiety. He knew he was going to heaven but the actual experience of dying frightened him so. I would tell him, "Please, Dad, don't be afraid. I will make sure you are comfortable. I won't leave you." Dad took my hand and kissed it and tearfully said, "Thank you, Judy, for being here." When he was actively dying, I kept saying through tears, "Dad, you will be able to see again. You will see Jesus! Go to Jesus. Don't be afraid. I love you, Dad."

When Dad stepped joyously into heaven, Mom was right where Dad wanted her, by his side, in their home. I collapsed on his chest and wept severely, wanting to go with him. One day, Dad, our adventures will begin again. What a glorious day that will be!

Come to me, all of you who are weary and carry heavy burdens, and I will give you rest. Take my yoke upon you. Let me teach you, because I am humble and gentle at heart, and you will find rest for your souls. For my yoke is easy to bear, and the burden I give you is light. Matthew 11:28-30

The ultimate joy is found in Revelations 21:4- *He will wipe every tear from their eyes, and there will be no more death or sorrow or crying or pain. All these things are gone forever.*

References and Suggested Readings

Alexander, Eben, M.D., *Proof of Heaven*, Simon &
    Schuster, Inc., NY, NY, 2012

Alfelt, Donnette R., *Comfort and Hope for Widows and
    Widowers*. Fountain Publishing, Rochester, MI, 2004

Andersen, Margaret L. and Howard F. Taylor, *Sociology:
    Understanding a Diverse Society, Third Edition.*
    Wadsworth, a division of Thomson Learning, Inc.,
    Belmmont, CA, 2004

Balk, David and Carol Wogrin, Gordon Thornton, David
    Meagher, *Handbook of Thanatology*. Association of
    Death Education and Counseling, The Thanatology
    Association, 2007

Boulay, Shirley Du, *Changing the Face of Death: The
    Story of Cicely Saunders,* Religious and Moral
    Education Press, Norwich, Norfolk, 2001

Brehony, Kathleen A., *Ordinary Grace*. Riverhead
    Books/Penguin Putnam, Inc., 1999

Brooke, Jill, *Don't Let Death Ruin Your Life*. DUTTON,
    member of Penguin Putnam Inc., NY, NY, 2001

Burpo, Todd, *Heaven is for Real,* W Publishing Group,
    imprint of Thomas Nelson, Nashville, TN, 2010

Callanan, Maggie and Kelley, Patricia, *Final Gifts*. Bantam
    Book, NY, NY, 1997

Coleman, William L., *When Someone You Love Dies.*
    Augsburg Fortress, 1994

Corr, Charles A., Clyde M. Nabe, Donna M. Corr, *Death
    and Dying, Life and Living, Fourth Edition.*
    Wadsworth, a division of Thomson Learning, Inc.
    Belmont, CA, 2003

DeHennezel, Marie, *Intimate Death: How the Dying Teach Us
    How To Live*. Alfred A. Knopf, Inc. 1997

DeSpelder, Lynne Ann and Albert Lee Strickland, *The
    Last Dance: Encountering Death and Dying, Seventh
    Edition.* McGraw-Hill, NY, NY, 2005

Duda, Deborah, *A Guide to Dying at Home with Dignity.* Aurora Press, 1987

Edward, John, *Crossing Over.* Jodere Group, Inc., San Diego,CA, 2001

Eldercare U.S. Department of Housing and Urban Development451 7th Street S.W., Washington, DC 2041, phone- (202) 708-1112 TTY: (202) 708-1455

Fearheiley, Don, *Angels Among Us: Amazing True Stories of Ordinary People Helped by Extraordinary Beings.* Avon Books, Inc., 1993

James, John W. and Russell Friedman, *The Grief Recovery Handbook.* Harper Collins Publishers, Inc., NY, NY, 1998

Johnson, Elizabeth A., *As Someone Dies.* Hay House, Inc.,Carlsbad, CA, 1995

Kirven, Robert H., *A Book About Dying.* Chrysalis Books,West Chester, PA, 1997

Kubler-Ross, Elisabeth, *Death: The Final Stage.* Simon & Schuster, Inc., NY, NY, 1975

Kubler-Ross, Elisabeth, *On Death and Dying.* Macmillian Publishing Company, NY, NY, 1969

Kubler-Ross, *Working It Through.* Macmillan Publishing Company, NY, NY, 1982.

Levine, Stephen, *A Year to Live: How to Live This Year As If It Were Your Last.* Bell Tower, 1997

Lung, Judith, *The Angels of God: Understanding the Bible.* New City Press, 1997

Lutzer, Erwin W., *One Minute After You Die.* Moody Pres,Chicago, IL., 1997

Morgan, Earnest, *Dealing Creatively with Death.* Zinn Communications, Bayside, NY, 1994

Morris, Virginia, *Talking About Death Won't Kill You.* Workman Publishing Co., 2001

Nuland, Sherwin B., 1994. *How We Die: Reflections on Life's Final Chapter*, Alfred A. Knopf, Inc., NY, NY, 1994

Palmer, Greg, *Death: The Trip of a Lifetime.* San Fran Harper Collins, 1993

Piper, Don, *90 Minutes in Heaven*, Fleming H Revell, division Baker Publishing, Grand Rapids, MI, 2004

Raspberry, Salli and Carole Rae Watanabe, *The Art of Dying.* Celestial Arts, 2001

Saunders, Cicely, *Beyond The Horizon*, Darton, Longman and Todd Ltd, London, SW, 1998

Singh, Kathleen D., *The Grace in Dying: How We Are Transformed Spiritually As We Die.* San Fran Harper Collin, 1998

Sparrow, G. Scott, *I Am With You Always: True Stories of Encounters with Jesus.* Bantom Book, 1995

Sykes, Nigel with Polly Edmonds and John Wiles, *Management of Advanced Disease,* Arnold Publishers, London, UK, 2004

The FORUM, Association for Death Education and Counseling, Vol.33, Issue 4, October, 2007

Webb, Marilyn, *The Good Death: The New American Search to Reshape the End of Life.* NY Doubleday, 1999

Resources:

American Association of Retired Persons/AARP
1-888-687-6677; http://www.aarp.org/families/grief_loss/

Association for Death Education and Counseling
http://www.adec.org/

Hospice Association of America (202) 546-4759
http://www.nahc.org/haa/

Hospice Directory- locate a hospice in the USA or
Canada at http://www.hospicedirectory.org/

Hospice Foundation of America
http://www.hospicefoundation.org/

International Association of Hospice and Palliative
Care http://www.hospicecare.com/

National Prison Hospice Association
http://www.npha.org/

Parents of Murdered Children 1-888-818-POMC
http://www.pomc.com/

Survivors of Suicide
http://www.survivorsofsuicide.com/index.html

The National Hospice and Palliative Care
Organization
http://www.nhpco.org/templates/1/homepage.cfm

About the Author

Judy Voss has been a Registered Nurse since 1973. She held certifications in Hospice and Palliative Care Nursing, in Thanatology/The Study of Death and Dying, and Health Education. While working for a hospice in Central Florida for over a dozen years she authored/co-authored three books that contained compilations of end-of-life stories. Her other books are of Biblical fiction, titled *Two Boys From Bethlehem* and *A King and his Camel*. Her Biblical fiction short story, *A Woman at the Cross,* follows next as a bonus read and is also available on amazon kindle. You can purchase *Finding Joy in Sorrow* on amazon.com or order through your local bookstore. The author welcomes your comments and can be reached via email at judyvosser@gmail.com

Just as a butterfly leaves its cocoon so too will I leave my earthly body, my spirit soaring to places I can only imagine.
Judy Voss

The following is the author's fictional rendition of an end-of-life story that was first told over 2,000 years ago.

A Woman at the Cross

I am a scorned woman. So why am I here sitting on this cold barren hill at the foot of the cross, huddled by his mother Mary knelt in prayer, and his disciple John? I have had many heartbreaking hours to figure out *why me* as we await Jesus' death.

A desperate shout out comes from the cross to my right so I rear my head up from my crouched position and glance over Mary's shoulders to John. His silhouette is barely visible in the dark of the night, which oddly should be in the light of the day. "What did he say, John?" My voice is shaky as the words pass through my trembling lips.

"I think he said *Why not save us and yourself?*"

A cry out is heard from the cross bearer on the left.

"And the other one?" I ask.

John shrugs and hangs his head low as the pitch from the jeering crowd behind us rises, hurling insults at the Messiah.

"Sir, what did he say?" I inquire loudly to the centurion, who stands brazenly three feet in front of me and an arm's length from Jesus' cross.

The man wraps his knuckles around the handle of his sword, then hesitantly turns his cheek toward me. In a harsh voice, he says, "For some reason, that scoundrel Dismas," the centurion points to the cross on the left, "says your friend has done nothing wrong."

Disheartened, I blurt out, "He IS right! He HASN'T!" In my attempt to stand, I catch my toes on my tunic hem and somehow, surprisingly, plant my feet solidly on the ground next to the Roman. "Sir?" I scrunch my nose up at the stench emitting from his heavily fortified body.

"Be VERY careful what you say, woman!"

Bile creeps up into my throat and I struggle to swallow it down. I look square into his eyes, then raise my prayerful hands to him. "Please, sir, have mercy on him! Please!"

NO mercy!" He abruptly turns and pushes against both my shoulders. "Not my fault he pretended to be the King of the Jews! Herod is the King!" he growled at me. The flicker of a torch reveals a jagged scar from his earlobe to his lip and, shockingly, he fingers it with a tenderness not becoming of him.

Defeated, I stumble back on the stark earth of Golgatha, grateful to see Joanna, Salome and other followers of Jesus close by. I sit cross-legged next to Mary, tuck my tunic between my legs, and weep softly. Taking her tiny prayerful hands in mine, I kiss them gently and raise them to my cheek. "I don't know how much more he can bear, Mary." I look to John with raised brows and tears flood my eyes, "Where's Peter and the others? Why aren't they here, John?"

The disciple scouts the area behind him, sadly nods, then looks upward to the Messiah.

Jesus returns John's gaze and through his bloodied and cracked lips says, "John, here is your mother."

John puts his arm around Mary and says, "Yes, Jesus, yes."

Despite the horrific sights ahead of me, the jeering mob at the crest of the hill, and the wailing mourners huddled nearby, I cannot stay focused on the here and now. I release Mary's hands and recall the day I first met her son and her.

It was a typical Magdala day, slightly overcast with the morning fog lifting off the Sea of Galilee. From the stoop of my family's courtyard, I watch fishing boats bob up and down in the distance as they skim across the water. My protective mother steps to my side and wraps her fingers around my slender wrist when she spots a handful of unknowns approach us. My heart pounds in my ears, I break out in a cold sweat, and start to shake in anticipation of what the demons inside of me are about to say and do!

The leader, dressed in a plain ankle length tunic, smiles broadly through his deep brown beard as he nears. He nods to my mother then stops just inches in front of me, laying both hands on my shoulders. His smile disappears and in a stern voice he says, "Get out of her! Demons! Get out!" They fought fiercely to stay but he would not allow it! "Get out, I command you! Leave Mary!"

What a glorious moment that was! Only those possessed, and obviously this man, know that I had no control over the appalling things the demons spewed out of my mouth: the belittling of my neighbors and strangers, the insults razed to the women in our town, and the taunting of innocent children. But I know emphatically, the whispers of me with men are all lies! Lies told by men whose advances I refused and so their lies about *Mary from Magdala* salvaged their egos, and gossip spread like wildfire. I often wonder how long the unjust accusations will follow me in life.

A screeching shout from the criminal on the cross to my right startles me back to the present. Mother Mary grabs my hands and sobs deeply. She rests her head on my shoulder, her scarf hangs low over her brows. I look to John who openly sobs. Mentally, I must escape the horror of the crucifixion, even if only briefly, so I return to that glorious day in Magdala.

As quickly as Jesus came, he went, and where his footsteps had just planted stood a woman. She was petite, and very pretty, looking at me with such kind eyes and a beautiful smile. I look at her with questioning eyes. Ever so lovingly, she takes my hands in hers, and kisses them. She tells me her name is Mary and her son, the healer, is Jesus.

We welcome Mary into our home, talk about our lives and she hers. She shares her son's message that we are to love one another, the forgiving of our sins, and life eternal. Awed by what she said, I realized my place is with her, and with him, and that is what I told Mary. She invites me to spend a few days in Capernaum with her and Jesus, meet some of his followers, and hear from Jesus himself. And that is what I did.

Since that day, near three years ago, Mary and I walked many miles side by side, following Jesus from one Galilean village to another, in Samaria, and into Jerusalem. The two of us cooked many meals, washed clothing, laughed, danced, sang, and slept in the same makeshift tents. Often, several other ladies who are followers of Jesus would join us. Mary had such a passion for the women in the villages. They could speak freely and question her apart from their spouses or other men. She loved to tell stories about Jesus, especially about his birth, and she loved being near him. What wonderful memories I have with my friend Mary. Something comes to mind, the premonitions she shared about her son, most often the same ones he conveyed, as well.

A commotion startles me out of my recollections as crucifiers laugh and shout hoorahs as they gamble away Jesus' clothing. My whole body shudders as I look to Jesus with a dread of the imminent, and pray to the God in heaven, "Dear God, have mercy on him!" Everything, the prayerful cries of Jesus' anguished followers, the pleading for mercy from the one hanging on his left and the other on his right, and a mother's weeping for her son who has endured pain beyond measure has brought me near to my breaking point. As the dark haze lingers heavily on the hilltop, I squint at each of the cruel faces of the crucifiers. I look up into Jesus' face and, finally, I admit to myself how fortunate I am to have been scorned. There is no place I would rather be than with him and his mother.

A voluminous scream of pain from Dismas sends dread deep into my gut. I focus my attention on the Messiah, my Savior. The thorns rest askew on his head and his bearded chin lies still in the curve of his neck. Dark blood slowly drips out of his wounds, splatting at the foot of his cross. His body is slumped downward, gruesomely supported by the four rusted spikes. Yet, somehow, Jesus lifts his head, eyes the heavens, and shouts out, "My God, my God, why have you forsaken me?" He eases his head down from whence it came.

My heart breaks and my arms ache to comfort him. My pulse quickens as I watch his eyelids flutter, then he ever so slowly opens them. He longingly looks down at the three of us as if to say I am so thankful you are here with me. As his lids slowly close, a deep, deep grumble begins in the bowels of the earth, then the ground heaves upward and outward, shaking me to my core. Wretched screams fill the dank air and soldiers frantically wave their arms as if dancing in their struggle to remain upright. The accusers and naysayers trip and tumble over each other as they dash down the hill to escape the wrath from deep below. I hold Mary as tightly as I can, and she me, and John both of us, and pray that this horrific tragedy ends.

Ever so slowly, a welcome respite comes as Golgotha gradually stills, the clamoring noises fade, and the sun begins lighting up the skyline. Then woefully, Jesus speaks again, his final words. "It is finished."

I gradually loosen my grip on Mary and knowingly look up to him, my eyes open wide in disbelief. His mother collapses prostrate on the shaken land, as does John. For me, all I wanted to do was touch Jesus. I boldly stand, fists clenched, and scream out, "NO!" I dart without hesitation to the cross, where no soldier should dare stop me, and embrace the wooden frame, and Jesus. With my face buried at the bend of his knees, I wail deeply. "NO, JESUS, NO!" A gut-wrenching awareness hits me that these brutal humans, who I shudder to call that, have murdered the one I love, the one so many love. The one we believed was going to save us all.

The scar-faced soldier grabs my sleeve and yanks me backward just as my scarf snags on a rusty, bloody nail and hangs haphazardly from the foot of the cross, my long brown hair draping my shoulders. I push the soldier away with a strength I didn't know I had and turn my attention back to Jesus. I tenderly rest my hands on his feet by the nail and lovingly release the edge of my torn scarf. Ever so calmly, I wrap my head with my scarf, step around the soldier, and take my seat next to my dearest friend, Mary. She is the one who held Jesus first, cared for him the best, and loved him the most. I engulf her in my arms, resting my face deep in the crevice of her neck. "Mary, dear Mary!" I weep uncontrollably as she lays her hand upon my head. She comforts me as a child, swaying back and forth, rocking our sorrows away as best she can, while loud crashing noises roar up from the holy city below as it shakes apart.

The scarred centurion lifts his sword from its holster, tosses it to the ground, and with certainty avows, "Surely, this man is innocent!"

The neighing of a horse and heavy stomping of its feet sends terror down my spine. I look up and see a Roman captain holding a spear high in the air above Jesus. Pulling my scarf low over my eyes, I shudder in dread at what his intent is. He taps Jesus' cross and hollers out in a booming voice, "Get him out of here!"

Soldiers kick up dust as they quickly rally around Jesus' cross, several position a ladder behind the center of the crossbeam, and another grabs a hammer from off a pile of rusty nails. Dowdy garbed funerary men scramble to the side of the cross who, no doubt, have been instructed to take Jesus to a rubbish heap.

"STOP!" shouts an onlooker who fervently rushes to the horseman and holds a sheet of papyrus high in the air. "I have permission from Pilate to care for him!" The soldiers halt all their movements and look to their leader for direction.

The captain leans forward over his saddle horn, snatches the paper from the claimant, and skims it quickly. "So be it! Be quick, as another is waiting!" He waves the soldiers away, turns his stallion, and returns from hence he came. The dowdy ones scamper away like river rats.

Mother Mary watches as John approaches the man entrusted to Jesus and says, "I want to help you. I am John, a disciple of Jesus."

"Yes, of course. I am Joseph, and this is Nicodemus."

Nicodemus begins his ascent up the rickety ladder when the scar-faced centurion steps to him. "Sir, it would be my honor to assist you with the holy one."

"Of course, we would be grateful."

Together, the four work in synchrony as they lovingly wrap linens around Jesus' arms, about his waist, and behind his knees, each overwhelmed with grief and aghast at the torture Jesus endured.

The centurion hands the hammer up to Nicodemus, then steadies the ladder for him while he precariously stands on the highest rung. As each of the nails are gently removed, Jesus is reverently lowered into the arms of Joseph and John, then joined by Nicodemus and the soldier.

I take Mary's hands and help her rise. We walk to a clearing on the hill away from the crowd, where we ease down onto a barren spot. Overcome with immense grief, we both cry unashamedly as we watch and wait.

The men move very slowly as they humbly carry Jesus to his mother and lay him down with his head resting in her lap. John sits by her side and I at his feet. I watch tearfully and sob openly, placing my hand over my mouth, as Mary ever so gently releases the crown of thorns from his bloody scalp and places it to her side. She kisses the torn flesh on his forehead and dabs his facial wounds with the hem of her favored scarf.

I watch as a stranger, carrying a bucket, approaches Mary and sets it next to the thorns, water sloshing overtop its brim onto the thorned crown.

John removes his waist cloth from his blood-stained tunic and dips it in the water. After squeezing the excess out, he places it in Mary's hands. She tenderly wipes his eyes and brows, his lips and face, and then his beard.

She slowly and reverently cleanses the dried blood from her son's severely battered and broken body as she weeps over him. I continue to watch in awe as Mary rinses the cloth again and again until her son is cleansed. She then hands the cloth back to John, who wraps it around his waist. Nicodemus hands John a jar of spiced ointments and, together, he and his mother apply the salve to Jesus' torturous wounds, then bind linens securely to his body. With Jesus' body nearly prepared for burial, Mary bends to her son's ear and whispers words no one else can hear. Then, sobbing, she collapses onto his chest.

Solemnly, the one who announced his authorization to care for Jesus, steps very slowly to Mary. His robe, heavily stained with the blood of the Messiah, displays one of wealth, made of fine silk and delicately embroidered. He kneels at the head of Jesus, holds his long gray beard close to his chest, and waits in stillness for Mary's acknowledgement. The Pharisee Nicodemus stands behind the elder, who I recognize as a trusted friend and follower of Jesus.

We all wait silently in our grief as Mary holds her son. She slowly lifts her upper body and rests back on her heels, her folded hands settle on her lap. She exhales deeply through pursed lips then looks from the face of her son to the kneeling man.

"I am Joseph, one who believes your son is truly the Messiah. I live in a town just outside Jerusalem, called Arimathea. With your approval, of course, Pilate has given me permission to place him in my tomb which is very near." He turns his head to the man behind him, then looks back to Mary. "This is my dear friend, Nicodemus, who also believes deeply in the teachings of Jesus. Perhaps you have met him before?" Mary nods slightly.

Mother Mary looks to me then back to Joseph. "Mary and I would like to go with you to see where he will lie."

"Yes, of course." Joseph motions to the man who presented the cleansing water. "Come forward, Barnum." We silently watch as he leads a donkey pulling a simple cart up to our gathering. I thought, how welcome are the familiar sounds of the donkey's bray and creaking wheels of the cart.

Together as one, we tenderly lift Jesus. I raise up his feet, Mary gently cradles his head in her hands, and the men cautiously balance his weight as we step to the small wagon. We lay Jesus on a bed of straw readied for him. From the corner of the cart, Nicodemus reaches for a beautifully embroidered blanket, and hands it to Mary. Lovingly, she lays the blanket across her son for his journey to the tomb.

With Barnum leading the donkey, we begin our descent down Golgotha. John supports a weakened Mary, his arm tucked around her tiny waist, as they follow steps behind Jesus. Joseph and Nicodemus follow behind the mother and son. I lag in the background and look around for Peter and the other disciples, wondering why they aren't here with Jesus.

After spotting the tomb in the distance, I am reminded of Eremos Cave, tucked in the hillside above the Sea of Galilee. Jesus loved to go there to pray. Mary and I loved it there, too, and it was only a short hike from Capernaum. I step quickly to Mary and tuck my arm under hers. She looks so lovingly to me, eyes flooded with tears, and smiles so sadly.

Barnum slows the donkey until the wooden wheels align with the tomb entrance. Several Roman soldiers wait in lazy repose on the grassy area, their shields lying within arm's reach. The men gently lift Jesus and carefully stoop through the low entrance as they carry him into the tomb. Mary and I wait outside as they complete his preparation for burial and spend their last moments with Jesus.

Upon them stepping out, I take Mary's hand and we bend down slightly as we enter the tomb. Kneeling side by side on the cold stone by Jesus, we speak not a word to each other. With my tears near spent and my emotions raw, we pray in silence. I ask God to care for Jesus and thank him for all he taught me, and for my healing. I slowly rise and step out of the tomb, leaving Mary with her son.

A soldier rolls from his side to his knees then stands. He tugs his breast plate down, yawns broadly, then steps firmly in front of Jesus' followers. "Times up! She's been in there long enough!"

John enters the tomb and returns with Mary, her hand resting on his arm. She has a calmness in her face and a look of peace that awes me. She walks to me and hugs me tightly, then turns and stares in silence as the soldiers approach the tomb.

Three of Herod's men pant and push and grunt while rolling an enormously large stone in front of the tomb entrance. "That's it! Go on!" one shouts out. "There is no more reason for you to be here."

With heartfelt goodbyes said, Nicodemus and Joseph head toward Jerusalem, with Barnum and his donkey following behind. John gently takes

Mary's hand and heads in the opposite direction. I linger behind in confusion and loneliness, watching as my dear friend walks away. I turn and glimpse at the tomb, wondering why, with all the amazing miracles Jesus performed, why didn't he save himself?

For near three days, I have anxiously waited to return to Jesus' tomb, busying myself in my friend's house while crying without ceasing. I am certain Salome will be glad when I head back to Magdala as I have swept her courtyard countless times, washed clean clothes, and reused dirty dishes. I have hauled so much water from the well there are no vessels left to fill. Most importantly, I have lovingly prepared spices and ointments to add to Jesus' linens. What I need now is for the sun to rise and Salome to waken!

I pull the heavy cloth away from the window and glance out. I don't spot any glimmer of light on the horizon but a rooster's crow in the distance alerts me to the time. I call out to Salome, "Wake up Salome, we must go!" She rises from her mat tucked in the far corner of her home and readies quickly.

With my spices and ointments secured in my apron and my torn scarf wrapped tightly around my head, I cautiously step out into the chill of the morning, with Salome behind me. I look to the east and, thankfully, see a dot of light skimming the skyline. As I turn back to the pathway that leads to Jesus' tomb, I hear Joanna shout out, "Hey, wait for us!" I smile at her and Mary of Clopas who have so selfishly provided sustenance for Jesus and his disciples.

The four of us walk briskly to the tomb, me leading the way. I breathe heavily and my palms start sweating as nerves set in, worried that the soldiers won't let us in Jesus' tomb.

Finally, I see it. *What's happened? How can it be?* The stone has been rolled away! I raise my tunic to my knees and run like the wind, leaving Salome, Mary, and Joanna in the dust. In my rush to enter the tomb, I fail to stoop low enough and scrape my scarf on the top sill. I quickly grab it as I stumble to where Jesus lay. "WHERE IS HE?" I scream out! In disbelief, I pick up the scented linens and scan fully the darkness of the tomb. *He is not here!* Dropping the burial cloths onto the stone bed, I rush out of the entrance and bump into the others as they are about to enter. "HE's NOT HERE!"

"How can that be, Mary?" Salome pushes pass me to where Jesus had lain. "Are you certain this is the right tomb, Mary?"

"Yes, yes, of course I am!" I drop my face into my hands and sob, "Where is he?"

"We must tell the others!" Salome says, as a look of dread washes across her face. She flees in panic, with the other women at her heels, leaving me alone in the empty tomb.

I am flabbergasted beyond understanding. I don't know where to go or what to do. Where should I look for Jesus? I step outside to ensure that, without question, this is the right tomb. There are no soldiers laying on the grassy knoll, and no one there to question.

"Mary! Mary!" I hear a familiar shout out in the distance and, while shading my eyes from the morning sun, I spot John sprinting toward me with Peter trailing behind. John stops in front of me, bends at the waist with his hands on his knees, gasping for air. "Is it true, Mary?"

Peter nearly knocks John over as he jogs by him, runs into the tomb, and returns as quickly as he entered, "WHERE IS HE?" he hollers out. John rushes to the entrance and glances in.

"I don't know, I just don't know!" I cry out. "Where would they have put him?"

Peter says, "We must find him!" Then I watch the two disciples rush away as quickly as they came.

Alone again, then suddenly I am startled by a flash of a very bright light streaming from the grave's entrance. Pushing my scarf further back on my head, I cautiously approach the tomb. I am in wonder of it all and peek inside. Two angels sit near where Jesus had lain, each dressed in brilliant white, and look directly at me. I stare with wide eyes and am bewildered at their presence.

The one closest to me speaks, "Don't be afraid." He looks to where Jesus had lain. "Why do you look for the living among the dead?"

They wait for me to answer, as I weep softly. "I, I don't know where they have taken him." I whisper, "Do you know?"

"Remember what Jesus of Nazareth told you? He said he would rise again," the other angel says. "So, there is no need to cry."

Suddenly, the angels fade away. I step in awe to where each of them sat, placing my hands on the cold, barren stone. I repeat the angel's words very distinctly, "He said he would rise again." Then, in slow motion, I turn and step into the morning sun. My sorrow over Jesus' absence is now conflicting with my exultation about his rising from the dead. I weep from the depths of my soul, as I carefully retrace my steps back to Salome's home.

I move to the side of the narrow way when I see a stranger approach. He stops and asks, "Why are you crying?"

I dab my eyes with the edge of my scarf, turn and point to Jesus' tomb a stone throw behind me. "Kind, sir, do you perhaps know where they have taken the one that was in that tomb?"

"Mary," he says.

Very slowly, I turn back with a slight hint of recognition in his voice. I look into his kind and compassionate eyes and am beside myself with excitement. "It is you, JESUS! You are ALIVE!" I drop to my knees at his feet in adoration, my sorrow replaced with an abounding joy, as he has truly risen.

It is nearly incomprehensible to me that Jesus chose to die, to save all of us, intentionally not calling a legion of angels to rescue him. I think back now on all his teachings, his parables, his Sermon on the Mount, his feeding of thousands, his healings, forgiving of our sins, and life after death. I could go on and on. He told us, his followers, so much without us comprehending it at the time. But what I remember most vividly and am most thankful for is the day in Magdala when he healed me, the scorned woman. Because if he hadn't done that, I would have never been the one sitting next to his mother at the foot of his cross.

Made in the USA
Columbia, SC
22 June 2023

18676907R00117